Praise for *A Parent*

MW00424626

"Pediatric cancer is a serious topic that demands clear-eyed and informed guidance. *A Parent's Guide to Childhood Cancer* delivers both a comprehensive review of what a cancer diagnosis means for a family and an easy-to-follow manual for supporting a child's healing journey. This is the first book to combine conventional and integrative medical approaches to treating pediatric cancer into one powerful resource. *A Parent's Guide to Childhood Cancer* is practical, empowering, and most of all, inspiring."

—BETH LAMBERT, co-author of *A Compromised Generation* and *Brain Under Attack*; founder of Epidemic Answers and Documenting Hope

"*A Parent's Guide to Childhood Cancer* is a vital integrative cancer guide for parents confronting the challenging reality of a child's cancer diagnosis. Dagmara Beine not only provides practical, easily digestible knowledge and guidance on integrative therapies and approaches but also instills a profound sense of hope and empowerment."

—IVELISSE PAGE, co-founder and executive director of Believe Big Institute of Health

"We're so, so proud of Dagmara Beine for writing the book that *needed* to be written! Nothing even close to this existed when our son was diagnosed with cancer. Trying to figure out the integrative approach to childhood cancer and pouring through obscure studies definitely earns you the honorary 'momcologist' degree . . . The difference is that Dagmara went on to get an actual degree and to lovingly compile all of the information in one place, making it way easier on you than it was for us. Dagmara Beine has risen to be one of the best in a breathtakingly short amount of time, and we're so lucky to have her in the childhood cancer community."

—RYAN AND TEDDY STERNAGEL, founders of The Stern Method

"Having a child diagnosed with cancer is a horrific experience for any parent to endure. But it's made even more difficult by the almost complete lack of information and support for pediatric cancer treatments beyond the conventional medical approach. In this indispensable book, Dr. Beine provides a practical primer on integrative cancer therapies for children based on a metabolic framework of understanding the disease. I can't recommend it enough."

—CHRIS KRESSER, MS, L.Ac., founder of Kresser Institute; *New York Times* bestselling author

"It is imperative that the parents of children with cancer become an instrumental part of their child's health care team. Dagmara Beine has not only created a blueprint for doing this but also for navigating an impaired conventional healthcare system in such a way to include holistic healing modalities, with a lens on individualized treatment plans best suited for their child.

"Beine has walked the walk both as a parent and as a professional, and now she offers up pragmatic and sage advice for families. Her strategies are comprehensive yet doable, including insights such as pressing the pause button after receiving a cancer diagnosis, treatment preparation tips, advice on how best to build a top-notch team, a guide to lab interpretations, health impacts from environmental toxicants, nutritional guidance, cancer-specific recommendations, and more.

"This in-depth study on the integration of mainstream medical and integrative tools in the treatment of childhood cancer is a most urgently needed resource, not only for families dealing with the heartbreak of a child with cancer but for medical providers as well. The excellent news is this front-line healthcare warrior mom has done the heavy lifting, outlined in this reader-friendly book, letting parents know that they are not alone on this journey."

—MICHELLE PERRO, MD, DHom, co-author, *What's Making Our Children Sick?*; co-founder and CEO, GMOScience

"Thank you, Dagmara Beine for your courage, your knowledge, and your compassion in writing this amazing book. It not only offers hope, but also has the potential to make a difference and even save the lives of our youngest members of the worldwide family of cancer-affected people. *A Parent's Guide to Childhood Cancer* offers a wealth of knowledge, options, and practical advice for parents, along with a well-balanced respect for the necessity of mainstream treatments in child oncology. This book can help us navigate the artificial boundaries between evidence-based hospital care and experience-based holistic medicine and show that the approaches are not exclusive but complementary. I highly recommend all parents, friends, and medical professionals treating children with cancer to read this book!"

—HENNING SAUPE, MD, author of *Holistic Cancer Medicine*

A Parent's Guide to Childhood Cancer

A Parent's Guide to Childhood Cancer

Supporting Your Child
with Integrative Therapies
Based on a Metabolic Approach

Dagmara Beine, PhD, PA-C

Forewords by
Dr. Nasha Winters, ND, L.Ac., FABNO
Dr. Paul Anderson, NMD

Chelsea Green Publishing
White River Junction, Vermont
London, UK

Project Manager: Rebecca Springer
Developmental Editor: Brianne Goodspeed
Copy Editor: Deborah Heimann
Proofreader: Diane Durrett
Indexer: Arbor Indexing
Designer: Melissa Jacobson

Printed in Canada.
First printing May 2024.
10 9 8 7 6 5 4 3 2 1   24 25 26 27 28

Our Commitment to Green Publishing

Chelsea Green sees publishing as a tool for cultural change and ecological stewardship. We strive to align our book manufacturing practices with our editorial mission and to reduce the impact of our business enterprise in the environment. We print our books using vegetable-based inks whenever possible. This book may cost slightly more because it was printed on paper that contains recycled fiber, and we hope you'll agree that it's worth it. *A Parent's Guide to Childhood Cancer* was printed on paper supplied by Marquis that is made of recycled materials and other controlled sources.

Library of Congress Cataloging-in-Publication Data

Names: Beine, Dagmara, 1980- author. | Winters, Nasha, 1971- writer of foreword. | Anderson, Paul S. (Naturopath), writer of foreword.
Title: A parent's guide to childhood cancer : supporting your child with integrative therapies based on a metabolic approach / Dagmara Beine, PhD, PA-C ; forewords by Dr. Nasha Winters, ND, L.Ac., FABNO, Dr. Paul Anderson, NMD.
Description: White River Junction, Vermont : Chelsea Green Publishing, [2024] | Includes bibliographical references and index.
Identifiers: LCCN 2024000243 (print) | LCCN 2024000244 (ebook) | ISBN 9781645021599 (paperback) | ISBN 9781645021605 (ebook) | ISBN 9781645021612 (audiobook)
Subjects: LCSH: Cancer in children—Popular works. | Cancer in children—Alternative treatment—Popular works. | Cancer in children--Diagnosis—Popular works. | Integrative medicine—Popular works.
Classification: LCC RC281.C4 B44 2024 (print) | LCC RC281.C4 (ebook) | DDC 618.92/994--dc23/eng/20240301
LC record available at https://lccn.loc.gov/2024000243
LC ebook record available at https://lccn.loc.gov/2024000244

Chelsea Green Publishing
White River Junction, Vermont, USA
London, UK

www.chelseagreen.com

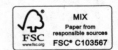

To my daughter, Zuza

Contents

Foreword

by Dr. Nasha Winters

I FIRST MET DAGMARA BEINE IN 2018 AT AN INTEGRATIVE MEDICINE symposium in Wichita, Kansas. I was there to give a presentation as a thirty-plus-year terminal cancer survivor, thriver, consultant, researcher, and teacher, as well as the co-author of *The Metabolic Approach to Cancer* and *Mistletoe and the Emerging Future of Integrative Oncology*. At that time, Dagmara's daughter, Zuza, was in remission from her diagnosis of acute myeloid leukemia (AML), and Dagmara was using that time to learn everything she could to help other families navigate the wilderness of cancer on a more holistic path.

Originally trained as a physician's assistant with experience in standard-of-care emergency medicine, Dagmara Beine's eyes, heart, and intellect were opened to the value of evidence-informed integrative therapies when Zuza (now twelve) was diagnosed with cancer at the age of three. Zuza's diagnosis, and the subsequent journey that she bravely embarked on with her mother to explore the very best of complementary care, has cast bright light on a better way forward for the treatment of childhood cancer. Although Zuza's path has been challenging and remains uncertain, she has already secured a profound legacy—inspiring change, education, and empowerment for families and childhood cancer patients around the world.

In pediatric cancer, the stakes are high. It can be extremely difficult for parents to not only understand available options, but to navigate conversations about these options with their child's medical team, family members, and concerned friends. Perceptions of integrative treatments vary widely, and skepticism often prevails for reasons including (but not limited to) a relative lack of scientific evidence, safety concerns (both legitimate and not), regulatory barriers, communication challenges, professional resistance, financial obstacles, and fear of delaying conventional treatment in order to fully explore various options (to name but a few).

The landscape is evolving rapidly, however, and there is increasing interest in integrative approaches among all stakeholders, including conventionally trained oncologists, especially when the approaches are evidence-informed and complement conventional care. There's good reason for this: The traditional model of cancer treatment resembles a battlefield, and the arsenal consists primarily of surgery, chemotherapy, and radiation. While these tools have saved lives, we cannot ignore the toll they take on the developing bodies, minds, and spirits of our youngest warriors.

Traditional cancer treatments are notorious for their harshness, leading to long-term effects that can compromise the child's future health and well-being, and requiring a careful balance between the imperative to eradicate cancer cells with the necessity to protect the child's overall health and future potential. Parents understand this, which is why so many of them seek out integrative therapies that can ease their child's suffering and promise to leave no stone unturned.

Indeed, the pursuit of comprehensive, integrative approaches is not only a scientific endeavor, but a moral imperative. Children, with their resilient spirits and burgeoning potential, deserve health-care approaches that not only combat illness, but will contribute to their overall and future well-being. Integrative medicine, which incorporates complementary therapies alongside conventional treatments, speaks to these intricate needs.

Moreover, the emotional toll on families navigating childhood cancer is immeasurable. Parents, already grappling with their child's devastating diagnosis, are often confronted with a maze of treatment options, each carrying its own set of risks and benefits.

The challenges of childhood cancer are real, but so is the potential for transformation and healing. The subsequent pages in this book will help parents navigate these complexities and transcend the many barriers, with coverage of personalized treatment plans, collaborative care models, evidence-based and evidence-informed research, all while emphasizing the importance of nutritional support, mind–body medicine, and patient and family empowerment. *A Parent's Guide to Childhood Cancer* also covers one of the most overlooked topics of all—holistic survivorship care.

Dagmara Beine empowers families with a comprehensive toolkit that extends beyond the confines of conventional treatments. The future of integrative pediatric oncology lies in this type of comprehensive, patient-centered, and evidence-informed approach. As awareness grows, research expands, and collaboration deepens, we anticipate a health-care landscape where integrative practices seamlessly complement conventional treatments, offering our youngest patients a more holistic and compassionate path toward healing. This book provides the roadmap.

Dagmara Beine's wonderful book is not merely a toolkit and a roadmap, however. It is also an impassioned call to action. It offers an invitation to collectively shape a future where the health and well-being of our children are at the forefront of medical practice. Driven by the conviction that healing should be as holistic as the beings we are striving to heal, Dagmara Beine has provided a beacon of hope in a landscape often clouded by fear and uncertainty. It is time for a paradigm shift—toward a more compassionate, personalized, and integrative approach. Dagmara and Zuza are leading the way.

I encourage you to approach these pages with an open mind, for within them lies the potential to change not only the way we perceive and treat childhood cancer, but also the very fabric of our health-care systems. The journey may be challenging, but the rewards are immeasurable, as we usher in an era where integrative medicine becomes an integral part of pediatric care, giving our children the foundation they deserve for a healthier, brighter, and more hopeful future.

With hope, dedication, and gratitude

to Zuza for being our teacher,

DR. NASHA WINTERS, ND, L.Ac., FABNO

Foreword

by Dr. Paul Anderson

I HAVE BEEN WORKING WITH PEDIATRIC CANCER PATIENTS AND THEIR families since the 1990s. In a recent book I wrote I made the statement, "A cancer diagnosis is bad, but having your child diagnosed with cancer is hell." I stand by that assertion.

Pediatric cancer is difficult on many levels, even when the child has positive outcomes. The process of diagnosis, treatment, care, and all that goes with it is unique. It is obviously a tough thing for the child and every family member, loved one, and caring friend.

In pediatric cancers the usual multi-layered issues of the cancer journey are magnified by many factors.

What I have learned to focus on is that, while a tough process, there are strategies that integrate standard cancer care and multiple other approaches that this integration can improve the overall care, outcomes, and quality of life for the patient and family.

In this book Dagmara Beine lays out multiple avenues available to the patient, family, and other caregivers to explore in this integrative process. These avenues include education about pediatric cancer, what to expect from standard therapies, integrative options, and much more. She brilliantly covers causes and aggravating factors, as well as how to address them. In my experience, standard oncology "knows" some factors (such as environmental toxicant exposure), but typically does not address them in the standard therapeutic approach. Beine walks her readers through these factors and offers real world tools to deal with them where appropriate.

This book is also personal. Beine and her family have been affected to the core by having a child with cancer. The level of information, help, and guidance from this perspective is not something that can be replicated.

I would highly recommend this book for anyone connected to or supporting a child who has cancer. It will help guide you through the difficult emotional processes, integration of standard therapies and other options, and give you options to consider that are often not discussed elsewhere. In my experience this information and approach leads to improved outcomes, better quality of life for the child, and better understanding for the parent and loved ones.

Dear reader, if you are using this book, you have a need that few people will truly understand, if they have not walked this road themselves. It is a tough road, and we may not get the outcome we want. Optimizing the care, and the cancer journey, for the child and everyone connected to the child, is crucial. This book can be your guide. There is added hope in being educated, assessing integrative approaches, and knowing you are doing all you can to support your child, or young loved one.

Strength and many blessings,

DR. PAUL S. ANDERSON, NMD

Introduction

My daughter, Zuza, was born on July 1, 2011. As a baby, Zuza didn't smile for a long time, and we joke that she still has the same crabby face she came into the world with. Most of her baby pictures show her eyebrows scrunched, almost as if she was contemplating what this human experience would be like. Along with her contemplative nature, she was also an incredibly sweet and easy baby. She slept well and loved spending time with her mom and dad. I remember fondly how she had little interest in learning how to crawl and we'd find her scooting around instead. She was doing things her own way—Zuza's Way.

When she was three years old, Zuza began to complain of leg pain. She lost her appetite and lost some weight. She started picking up frequent colds and would take longer to get over them. My husband, Ryan, and I both worked as emergency room physicians' assistants and between our combined medical experience and our parental intuition, we sensed that something serious might be wrong. We pressured Zuza's pediatrician to run labs.

On a Tuesday afternoon at the end of February in 2015, I found myself anxiously awaiting the phone call that would change our lives. Intuitively, I somehow already knew that nothing would be the same. I still remember the feeling in my body, like it already knew what my mind was about to learn. That morning I took my phone into the shower with me to be sure I wouldn't miss the call. Eventually, it rang and the pediatrician confirmed my fears.

The pediatrician told me that Zuza's lab test results were suggesting that she had acute lymphoblastic leukemia (ALL), a fast-moving cancer of the bone. ALL is the most common leukemia diagnosis in children. Because ALL progresses rapidly, we were advised to start Zuza on chemotherapy right away.

———

I'm sorry you're reading these words, because it most likely means that your child, like my child, is one of the thousands of children diagnosed with cancer every year. Maybe your child has just received a diagnosis and you feel like a tiny ship being tossed around on a stormy sea, desperate to make all the right decisions, not a single mistake that might result in more harm or suffering. Or perhaps your child is in the midst of treatment that seems as though it will never end. Your entire family has been in survival mode for months, or even years, and you are exhausted from the endless roller coaster of emotion—hope and despair—wondering with every decision and medical recommendation if you could be doing more, or better, for your child. Or maybe your child has achieved remission and you want—you need—to do everything in your power to make sure it stays that way. Whoever you are, I'm sorry you're here, because it likely means your child is going through something no child deserves. But I'm also glad you're here. I wrote this book for you.

I wrote this book to share everything I've learned in the past ten years with other parents who are supporting children through pediatric cancer. As of this writing, Zuza has attained five-year remission once and relapsed three times. She has gone through chemotherapy *many* times and undergone two bone marrow transplants. We have done conventional therapy on its own as well as combined with various integrative therapies. We have seen her suffer terribly through side effects such as mucositis and dangerous complications such as graft-versus-host disease. We have also watched her sail through serious treatments with almost no side effects or complications whatsoever, jumping on her trampoline within hours of being discharged from the hospital.

While we don't know whether Zuza will ultimately vanquish cancer, we do know what has prolonged or shortened her treatment, what has reduced her side effects, what has allowed her to return home to her own bed and family more quickly, what has spared her unnecessary and often toxic treatments for side effects, and what she has told us has made her feel better or worse. We've observed, studied, and consulted with world experts in the treatment of childhood cancer as well as experts in the most effective comprehensive integrative therapies. What I can tell you is this: With cancer, there is no silver bullet. But there is a better way than what conventional oncology will offer you.

This is the book I needed, and couldn't find, when Zuza was first diagnosed—as well as when she completed treatment, was struggling with side effects, relapsed, and even when she was feeling well but we were full of fear that soon she wouldn't be. If something positive can come from our own struggle, it will be that other parents have this information at their fingertips, without having to hunt for it or learn through trial and error over the course of months or even years and that it will inform your own advocacy and decision-making.

But my book also has a very specific angle. After nine years in this fight, I can say with some assurance that the biggest crisis in pediatric cancer is the lack of comprehensive medical support: the importance of nutrition, sleep, movement, and stress reduction; how to help your child's gut heal after chemotherapy destroys their microbiome; how to harness the power of epigenetic tests to inform individualized decisions for a chemotherapy regimen; how to safely manage side effects from conventional treatment or reduce the risk of complications; and much more. We'll delve into the cutting-edge science that questions the genetic origins of cancer and instead views it through the lens of metabolic and mitochondrial dysfunction. We'll also look closely at the powerful contributions of a new metabolic therapy: the ketogenic diet.

Nothing I write in this book is mutually exclusive with conventional treatment. I am not asking you to turn away from conventional treatment. The oncologists will know what chemotherapy to use, the surgeons will know what to cut out, the radiologists will know where to radiate, and the transplant doctors will know how to replace your child's immune system. Their immense knowledge is valuable; this is what they were trained to do, and many of them do it expertly.

However, your child's oncologist was not educated in nutrition, and your child's inpatient nutritionist is most likely developing your child's nutrition plans around what is on the formulary at your hospital. Your child's doctors did not receive lessons in medical school about the importance of gut healing beyond Pepcid and proton-pump inhibitors. This is not about who's to blame. It is about a better way to navigate the broken system that your child is now a part of. It is up to you to create a comprehensive team and comprehensive plans that will help your child thrive. This book will show you how.

The chapters in this book are organized in roughly the order that events tend to unfold, from initial diagnosis to post-treatment recovery, and according to the sorts of decisions you might be faced with, as a parent, at each stage and the sort of information that will be useful as you weigh those decisions. However, life is never that tidy and, in some cases, you might be making certain decisions simultaneously. For example, I have information on building your child's medical team in chapter 2, but you might be doing this at the same time as you are gathering additional data, which is covered in chapter 3. Every situation and every child is different, so there is no easy way around this. However, my goal has been to organize the book in such a way that the relevant material will be as accessible as possible to the overwhelmed parent. I've included four appendices with additional resources, menu-planning ideas, packing lists for inpatient treatment, and details on lab work and testing your child might undergo, for readers who want to go deeper.

———

Integrating functional therapies with conventional treatment doesn't guarantee sustained remission, but I believe it is a better way. That said, I have also witnessed my share of miracles: pediatric patients who came to me when there was "nothing more" that could be done, and with integrative therapies achieved complete remission. And with my own Zuza, while of course our goal is complete remission, I am still convinced that the incorporation of integrative medicine therapies has been a better way, even as the cancer has returned.

Using a comprehensive integrative approach does not guarantee a cure, but it does involve less suffering. It leaves no rock unturned, and it does, I believe, decrease the chance of relapse and late effects. For my patients who have thrived, it has never been just one thing. It is never just nutrition or just mistletoe or just a key supplement. It is truly individualized support. When every decision we made about supplements and therapies was individualized to Zuza's needs and conventional treatment, that was when she truly thrived.

CHAPTER 1

Stop and Breathe

MY DAUGHTER, ZUZA, WAS DIAGNOSED WITH ACUTE LYMPHOBLASTIC leukemia (ALL) in February 2015 when she was three years old. My husband, Ryan, and I were told that with immediate treatment, the survival rate for ALL was very good: 80 to 90 percent of patients with ALL will attain complete remission.

The day after she was diagnosed, Zuza began inpatient chemotherapy with vincristine. We were informed that she would likely have neuropathy as a side effect, and that it was a possibility that she would stop walking completely. We were overwhelmed, and though we were terrified, we were also happy to be told that, despite the toxicity of the treatment, it would make the cancer go away.

Several days into Zuza's treatment, however, Ryan and I learned that her diagnosis was incorrect. In fact, Zuza had acute myeloid leukemia (AML), a less common but more dangerous form of leukemia, with a five-year survival rate 20 to 30 percent lower than ALL. In addition to a worse prognosis, my now terrified three-and-a-half-year-old daughter had been receiving treatment that was not only making her sick with side effects, it wasn't even helping her recover from the kind of cancer she actually had.

The first of many cancer lessons Ryan and I learned the hard way is that misdiagnoses are not uncommon. But how were we supposed to know that? We were just two terrified parents who had never, ever been through anything like this before in our lives. We were scared, walking around in a daze, blindly stumbling through one appointment and telephone call after another. Even though Ryan and I were both medical professionals with decades of ER experience, we had no experience with childhood cancer or any other kind of life-threatening illness in our own child. All we had to go on at that point were doctors' recommendations. We were desperate for any kind of authority or certainty we could lean on.

Stop and Breathe

Because of Zuza's experience—as well as similar stories I've heard from many other families—my first recommendation, as both a parent and a medical professional, is when your child receives a cancer diagnosis: Pause.

I get it. You feel a sense of urgency. Every parent feels this way, which is why it is such a common mistake to rush into treatment. But in most cases, there is no need to start chemotherapy, radiation, or even surgery right away. The chances are good that this cancer has been developing for months or even years and, in most cases, a few more weeks of gathering your wits, collecting information, data, and second opinions, and making well-informed, intelligent decisions from a place of parental authority rather than panic will be a positive calculated risk in your child's prognosis.

That said, there *are* some circumstances where the tumor is growing in an area that creates a life-threatening situation and surgery must be performed immediately. I am not speaking about those situations. I am speaking about the majority of situations in which a child receives a cancer diagnosis and, before test results are even back, a child is unnecessarily rushed into treatment, sometimes as soon as the day after diagnosis.

In most cases, it is reasonable to ask your child's oncology team if it is possible to wait a few weeks so that you can take time to absorb this information and prepare your child for treatment. Politely explain that you want the results of all lab work, imaging, and biopsies to confirm diagnosis before starting treatment, as well as access to all data and information about the diagnosis that they are able to provide.

During this time, your child may need supportive care, such as IV fluids for dehydration or an antibiotic for infection. This is also a good opportunity to get to know your child's medical team, which will become a factor in not only your child's prognosis but your entire family's quality of life.

The other thing you should do during this time is pursue a second opinion. Every child deserves one. This will give you an important opportunity to learn more about the diagnosis and recommended treatment, give you confidence in the upcoming course of action, and help you understand what questions to ask. Most second opinions are done virtually with the assistance

Preparing for Treatment

When you step into the world of pediatric cancer, you are living in the world as it is, not the world as it should be. If your child is in a situation in which treatment must start immediately, before you have even wrapped your brain around your new life, don't despair. Here are a few simple recommendations to prepare for treatment, regardless of when your child begins.

- Protect your child's sleep. Teach them to wind down before bed with a meditation or a story.
- Spend as much time outside with your child as you can.
- Try to eliminate or at least reduce processed and artificial foods from your child's diet. Remove sugar and, ideally, grain, if possible; this is especially true if radiation is part of your child's protocol. If they have insulin resistance, the radiation will not work as well. Radiation needs preparation, both in making sure your child is metabolically flexible, with key supplements and herbs on board that will both protect healthy cells and make the radiation more effective. In most cases, I advise against starting radiation before you have an integrative oncology practitioner involved in your child's care.
- Give your child basic supplements, such as vitamin D3, zinc, magnesium, and omega fatty acids.

We will delve into all these topics in greater detail throughout the book. Ideally, you will have the time you need to absorb the necessary information and put it into practice. Preparation is extraordinarily helpful in minimizing stress, reducing drawbacks, and maximizing treatment benefit. But you may not have the luxury of preparing as much as you would like to, and that's OK. (If your child will be receiving inpatient treatment, see appendix C for a recommended packing list for both patient and caregiver.)

If you do nothing else, take some time—it could be three months, but it could also be twenty minutes—and be intentional about preparing emotionally, physically, and spiritually. If you are able, I recommend at least one parent, if not both, take time off to be at home with your child. Make that time off together sacred. Laugh, play, and snuggle. Remind your child how capable their body is of healing and give them your undivided time before they feel sick and separated from you in a hospital. Ask a few trusted people to make and deliver nutritious meals; ask someone else to start a fundraising page. Surround your other children with love and hope.

of your initial team and social worker. Most hospital websites include information about their second-opinion process.

Like the twenty-first-century parent you are, you will probably also be jumping on the internet to learn as much as you can and conduct some of your own research. This can be valuable, but caution is warranted. Be aware that most studies on the internet are behind the times or do not tell the whole story, and some are flat-out junk. It is easy to get freaked out by what you find on the internet. Especially when it comes to prognosis statistics, remember: Your child is not a statistic. Do not get hung up on statistics and prognoses; gather information specific to your child's diagnosis so that you can understand different options presented to you.

Pausing is one of your most important tasks during the window of time between diagnosis and the start of treatment—this pause is your opportunity to stop and take a breath. And another. And another. *Take* it. *Make* the space. Practice and learn how to do it, so you can return to that practice in the weeks and months to come. You are about to get on an emotional roller coaster unlike anything you've ever experienced. What's more, it could last for *years*. Resist the urge to call everyone you know or get on social media and shout your plight to the world. Maintain a protective circle around your child, yourself, and your family. If you have a partner, hold space for each other's (possibly different) reactions. Hold space for your child, your other children if you have them, and yourself. Create a space of peace within yourself and practice visiting it, especially when things feel chaotic around you.

Stop. Breathe.

Five years after Zuza's initial diagnosis, she relapsed. We were told—again, with great certainty—that it was treatment-related leukemia with such a poor prognosis that palliative care was her best option. A few weeks later, we found out that the diagnosis was incorrect. The difference the second time around? We didn't rush into treatment. In fact, we didn't start for more than a month. Ryan and I paused, gathered our wits, weighed our options, asked our questions, and *then* made the best decisions we could for Zuza. It made all the difference in the world.

Now, Get a Grip

When I say, "get a grip," I don't mean that in a disparaging or belittling way. Far from it. What I mean is that your life has just been turned upside down and inside out—very suddenly and most likely without warning. It is like you have been knocked off your feet by a huge blast you never saw coming. You are dizzy and disoriented and in shock, and trying to get back up on your feet.

This is your new life.

You will be living it for many months and, possibly, many years. Not only that, as a parent, you will need to be the rock solid foundation for your child—and possibly other children in your family, if you have them—as they navigate this new life.

That is a very big deal. Do not let the insane pace of twenty-first-century life—and twenty-first-century parenting—dictate what happens next. You need to allow yourself to get your bearings. This is not an overnight event; it is an ongoing process. And the reason getting your bearings matters so much right now is because it will set the tone and intention for the months and years to come.

What exactly *is* cancer? *Cancer* is defined as uncontrolled division of abnormal cells and the spread of those cells throughout the body.[1] As these abnormal cells grow and spread, they affect the rest of the body's organs.

The Fourteen Hallmarks of Cancer

Adapted from "Hallmarks of Cancer: New Dimensions" by Douglas Hanahan.[2]

1. Sustained proliferation: Cancer cells find ways to grow.
2. Insensitivity to antigrowth signal: Cancer cells learn how to evade growth suppressors.
3. Evasion of apoptosis: Cancer cells learn how to resist cell death.
4. Limitless replicative potential: Normal cells die after a certain number of divisions; cancer cells do not.
5. Inducing angiogenesis: Cancer cells create new blood supply to solid tumors to get the oxygen and nutrients they need to grow.
6. Activating invasion and metastasis: Cancer cells spread to other sites in the body.
7. Deregulated metabolic pathways: Cancer cells use an abnormal metabolism for energy and nutrients.
8. Evasion of the immune system: Cancer cells suppress immune cells and evade the immune system.
9. Cancer-promoting inflammation: Tumors activate an inflammatory response.
10. Genome instability and mutation: Cancer cells have an inability to repair DNA and production of mutated cells continues.
11. Nonmutational epigenetic reprogramming: Global changes in the epigenetic landscape are a common feature of many cancers.
12. Polymorphic microbes: Microorganisms can exert protective or deleterious effects on cancer progression, development, and response to therapy.
13. Senescent cells: Senescent cells can stimulate tumor development and malignant progression.

14. Unlocking phenotypic plasticity: Malignant cells evade differentiation and unlock what is known as phenotypic plasticity to allow the malignant cells to continue to grow. In other words, they can change their identity into something that is more inclined to proliferate.

This is a very basic description of what cancer is. However, there are different theories about *why* cancer cells grow out of control. Most current research and treatment protocols are based on the somatic theory of cancer, which is that cancer is caused by genetic mutation.[3] These mutations accumulate until they result in a tumor that must be removed to prevent metastasis and death. These mutations are considered random, so the only things a patient can do are surgery, radiation, or chemotherapy to remove the cancer. If your oncology team tells you that your child's cancer is just bad luck, they are basing this statement on the somatic theory.

The metabolic theory of cancer, on the other hand, looks at the cancer cell itself and its cellular environment. The origins of this theory trace back to Otto Warburg, who won the Nobel Prize in 1931 for discovering that cancer cells consume more glucose and produce more lactate than normal cells.[4] Normal, healthy cells have much less of a need for glucose. Therefore, if you limit glucose and dramatically decrease carbohydrates, you are limiting energy to cancer cells with potentially little effect on healthy cells.

Nearly a century later, Dr. Thomas Seyfried, a cancer researcher and professor of biology at Boston College, further developed the theory that cancer is a metabolic disease whose etiology (*cause*) is not primarily in the nucleus but is in the mitochondria, the energy factories of the cell. In this paradigm, oncogenes are the symptom of an underlying process, not the cause. Whereas conventional oncology treats cancer like a weed—doctors pull it (surgery) or treat it (with chemo or radiation) and hope it does not come back—the metabolic approach to cancer looks at the soil the cancer grew in.

Nuclear cell transfer studies back up the metabolic theory.[5] In these studies, researchers remove the nucleus (where the genetic information is stored) from a cancer cell and insert it into a healthy cell. If cancer is encoded in DNA, it would follow that the healthy cell would become cancerous. But in fact, the result is typically a healthy cell. And vice versa: If researchers remove a healthy nucleus and insert it into a cancer cell, it would follow that the cancerous cell would become healthy. But, in fact, the result is typically a cancerous cell.

There are a lot of legitimate questions about the somatic theory, and many well-respected researchers and clinicians consider cancer to be primarily a metabolic disease, not a genetic one. Indeed, *many* illnesses—including cancer, mental illness, Alzheimer's disease, diabetes, and much more—are increasingly investigated for their metabolic (often mitochondrial) origins, rather than their genetic origins. At the very least, the metabolic approach to illness offers a new lens through which to understand serious disease. At its most profound, it completely overturns the prevailing medical model of what cancer is and how to treat it.

Despite this developing understanding of cancer, most treatments—and research funding—remain based on the somatic theory.[6] Between 2003 and 2013, more than sixty-two new oncology drugs were approved, many targeting oncogenes. Of these, only 43 percent offered a survival benefit of three months or longer, and 30 percent offered no survival benefit at all.[7] Most improvements in cancer care result from increased ability to treat infections and acute care situations, and studies are often designed to measure tumor shrinkage, not survival or quality of life.

Through my extensive research, clinical practice as an integrative oncology practitioner, personal experience, and collaboration with experts in the field, I have arrived at the viewpoint that the etiology of cancer is a multifaceted matter, far from being definitively categorized, and is probably attributable to a synergistic interplay between somatic and metabolic theories.

Unfortunately, the somatic theory is the paradigm we're stuck in—for now. And, as the parent of a child with cancer, your options for refusing treatment for your child are fewer than they would be for yourself. (See "Legal Issues," page 22.) But there are many excellent integrative therapies based on the metabolic approach to cancer that can complement conventional cancer treatment. The reason I wrote this book is to share with you what I've learned about those integrative therapies.

As the parent of a child with cancer, you will need to get used to gathering information from both conventional and integrative oncology in order to make sound decisions. This is not easy, especially as you are unlikely to have expertise in either conventional oncology or integrative therapies. That is OK. Think of yourself as the general contractor: You may not know how to do everything, but you will assemble a team that does. Get used to asking questions, listening carefully to the answers, and integrating what you learn into your growing understanding of your child's illness and care. (See sidebar "The First Twelve Questions.")

The path ahead is not going to be easy. But you can do this. And you *will* do this because your child needs you to. That doesn't mean you have to be perfect, or that you have to know everything. You aren't and you don't. It means you have to journey forward into the unknown, gathering

The First Twelve Questions

1. What is my child's precise diagnosis?
2. How common is this diagnosis among children?
3. What is my child's prognosis?
4. Is this a fast-growing or a slow-growing cancer?
5. What treatment do you recommend?
6. What is the time frame for this treatment?
7. Is this treatment curative or palliative?
8. If this treatment does not cure my child's cancer, what happens next?
9. May I have a list of all medications and all known side effects of all medications involved in my child's recommended treatment?
10. Are you open to collaborating with an integrative oncology practitioner and a holistic nutritionist?
11. Can I refuse the treatment you are recommending? Can I refuse parts of it? What happens if I refuse parts or all of the treatment?
12. What do you think caused my child's cancer?

the best information you possibly can, to make the best decisions you possibly can.

Having lived in this world for years, having known countless families in this world, and having advised hundreds of patients in this world, I assure you that there are many unknowns. But there is one thing I do know with certainty: There is a better way than what conventional oncology has to offer. And the effort you put into navigating integrative therapies and approaches will be worth it. Your child is worth it.

Off we go.

CHAPTER 2

Build Out the Team

ONE OF YOUR FIRST STEPS WILL BE TO ASSEMBLE THE BEST POSSIBLE medical team that will integrate the best that conventional cancer treatment has to offer with the many other available therapeutic options, including nutrition, from integrative medicine. In order to do this, it is extremely important to understand the power and the limitations of conventional oncology. Conventional oncology sees cancer treatment through a deep, but narrow, lens—chemotherapy, radiation, surgery—and excludes some other important factors that will also influence your child's prognosis and quality of life. These factors include nutrition, stress, sleep, movement, and social support, as well as many powerful integrative medicines that run the range from highly safe and effective (and often used in mainstream oncology elsewhere in the world) to ineffective, wacky, and sometimes downright dangerous. Conventional oncology is not going to sort out these factors or integrative medicines for you. That's your job.

It's also essential for you to understand that the limitations of conventional oncology are, for the most part, not the fault of your child's medical team, the hospital, or anyone else directly involved in your child's care. It's much bigger than that. The problems with conventional oncology are systemic. They are related to insurance, standards of care, pharmaceutical companies, medical schools, state and federal laws, and much more. And it is a far more complex problem than you have the luxury of pretending you can solve. *Your* job is to support your child with every tool at your disposal, making the best decisions you possibly can on their behalf, within the context of a broken and sometimes corrupt system and a situation—childhood cancer—that no parent and no child should ever have to deal with. This is not a book about how things should be. This is a book about doing the best you can with how things are.

So buckle up. You are now the general contractor of your child's health. You are probably not an expert on their diagnosis and that's OK—because you will hire a team with the expertise you need. But never forget: You are in charge. You are the person who bears the ultimate responsibility. No one knows your child or loves your child more than you do. No one cares more than you do. You can do this. Here are the essentials of a good team.

Oncologist

You obviously want your child to have an oncologist with deep expertise in your child's diagnosis as well as a high rate of success in treatment. But it's not always so simple. Often an oncologist with decades of experience is your best bet, but it can also be true that less experienced oncologists are better versed in the latest and emerging research, not to mention highly motivated to prove themselves. You want someone who will take your questions and concerns as a parent seriously and who is willing to partner with an integrative oncology practitioner (see "Metabolic Oncology Practitioner" on page 19). If your oncologist seems skeptical of integrative support, it is most likely out of genuine concern for your child, lack of knowledge about the tools you wish to incorporate, and a fear of liability.

For example, certain supplements can get in the way of treatment; other supplements can improve treatment efficacy and mitigate side effects. Your child's oncologist will probably not know much about this, and they may respond that they need to see big, randomized studies on anything you want to incorporate into your child's treatment. Unfortunately, large, randomized studies are wildly expensive and most are funded with the goal of marketing pharmaceutical drugs. There are amazingly effective treatments that are "unproven" because they have not found a wealthy sponsor. It is likely that your child's oncologist will want to err on the side of few or no supplements during treatment.

The bottom line is that oncologists are extremely focused on medical oncology, not on deep nutrition and integrative therapies. Most have almost zero training in nutrition. Try to keep in mind that their intentions are good—they want your child to survive and thrive—and their concerns are valid. There is a lot of bad advice out there, and certain supplements and therapies can harm, not help, your child if not used properly. Bear all of this in mind. At the same time, do not allow the limitations of conventional oncology to force limitations upon your child's care and prognosis.

You also need to know that in some situations, a parent who does not comply with recommendations for conventional cancer treatment may be subject to child welfare involvement (see "Legal Issues" page 22), and this can depend, in part, on the oncologist you select. You do not want to risk having your child removed from your custody because of your medical decision-making. Ask as many questions as you need to ask until you have a solid handle on all likely scenarios.

Location is also a factor. If your child's diagnosis is relatively common and you have a good hospital nearby, in most cases it will make sense to use the local hospital rather than to travel. In fact, for certain common diagnoses, such as ALL, many hospitals utilize the same protocol. Don't underestimate the benefits of being close to home, such as home-cooked meals and family support.

If your child's case is rare or complicated, however, it might be worth traveling for the very best care. It might also make sense to travel for care if your child relapses and you want to work with the best team with acknowledged experts and the most up-to-date trials. It's always a trade-off, but for complex surgeries, new treatments, or uncommon diagnoses you may decide to travel so your child can be treated by the oncologist of your choice.

The Next Twenty Questions to Ask Your Child's Oncologist

1. Are you open to using nonpharmaceutical drugs for treating side effects? If not, why not?
2. What are the short-term side effects of the drugs used in the recommended treatment?
3. What are the long-term side effects of the drugs used in the recommended treatment?

4. Do any of these drugs have life-threatening side effects?

5. How old are the drugs you recommend? How long have they been around?

6. Are there additional drugs, like steroids or antibiotics, that my child might need to take?

7. What happens if my child gets a fever during treatment? (Can I refuse Tylenol?)

8. What is the recurrence rate after this treatment? Where does that statistic come from?

9. What is the five-year disease-free survival rate for my child's diagnosis with this treatment?

10. What is the five-year disease-free survival rate for my child's diagnosis if I do nothing?

11. How much does this treatment contribute to five-year survival for my child's cancer?

12. What is the risk that this treatment will make the cancer more aggressive?

13. Is this treatment carcinogenic?

14. Does this chemotherapy kill cancer stem cells?

15. What is the risk that this treatment will make the cancer cells more resistant to future treatment? What is the plan if that happens?

16. What other treatment options are available besides the one you are recommending?

17. What do you recommend my child eat while undergoing chemotherapy? Are there any foods that should be avoided?

18. Will you be ordering genetic testing to be sure the drugs will not be severely toxic to my child?

19. I will be ordering an epigenetic test. Can we use these results to modify treatment for my child?[1]

20. What if the treatment makes my child very sick? Can I refuse the continuation of treatment or the continuation of parts of treatment?

Metabolic Oncology Practitioner

Another essential member of your child's team is a medical professional with expertise in integrative therapies for cancer—ideally for children. This person might have a few different titles, for example, "integrative oncology practitioner" or "metabolic oncology practitioner." Regardless of the specific title, it is essential to identify an experienced clinician who can navigate the worlds of both integrative and conventional approaches to cancer treatment.

While there are many excellent integrative *general* practitioners, few of them have the knowledge and experience necessary to support your child through cancer. I recommend practitioners trained by the Metabolic Terrain Institute of Health, cofounded by Dr. Nasha Winters, which keeps an online directory of "terrain certified practitioners" that is searchable by location and specialty. (Full disclosure: I received my training and certification as a metabolic oncology practitioner through this program.)

Unfortunately, as of this writing, there are few integrative oncology practitioners who specialize in the treatment of *children*. There are many reasons for this, including the professional risk of treating children with life-threatening diseases using unconventional methodologies and the particular complications and considerations related to medical treatment for serious illness in children. (Consider, for example, how treatment might affect a child's future fertility versus treating an older adult who may have already had children— and many more considerations such as these.) This is unfortunate, because there are many children who would benefit enormously from this care, for whom it could make a difference in quality of life, or even in life versus death.

Finally, as in every field, there are people in the field of integrative medicine who pose as experts but are not. There are even those who may prey upon parents' desperation. This can present a huge risk to your child's health as well as drain your bank account and waste your time and precious energy. Ask every question you need to ask, seek referrals and recommendations, and remember that if a practitioner is not comfortable being grilled by a concerned parent, they may not be the person you want to trust with your child's health.

All of this is to say that it may take some time to find the right person with the skill and training you're looking for, as well as someone you and your child are comfortable with. I urge you to stay the course. (Many practitioners will do virtual visits, which means you don't necessarily need to work with someone who is within driving distance of your home.) This clinician can become an extremely valuable member of your child's medical team, offer a more comprehensive perspective of your child's overall health than conventional oncology alone does, and aid immensely in the difficult decisions you'll need to make as a parent. Ideally, this team member will take the whole child (and, in some cases, the whole family) into account.

This clinician may help you ask the right questions of your oncology team; help you identify an integrative nutritionist (see below) for your team; help evaluate the test results and a suite of integrative therapies suitable to your child's specific case; and offer support in managing side effects, healing the gut, and preventing recurrence or late effects. (Up to 95 percent of pediatric cancer survivors have late effects and multiple chronic life-threatening disease processes by age forty-five.[2]) A metabolic oncology practitioner may also be able to help you identify and address the underlying risk factors that may have contributed to the original diagnosis and develop nutrition and lifestyle changes that will be more supportive of the health and well-being of your entire family. And much more.

My experience—based both on my formal medical training and my daughter's initial cancer diagnosis—led me to believe so strongly in the value of this role that after Zuza's first battle with AML, I became a terrain certified practitioner myself and opened a clinic—Zuza's Way—primarily dedicated to the integrative medical support of children with cancer and their families. I speak from experience working with hundreds of families, as well as learning to support my own daughter with integrative therapies, when I say that the metabolic approach has the power to reduce suffering, improve quality of life, and improve prognosis and outcomes more than conventional oncology can alone.

Integrative Oncology Nutritionist

Another blind spot that you may discover in conventional oncology is its ambivalence toward nutrition. Most oncologists do not have training in nutrition and, unfortunately, most hospital nutritionists and dieticians focus on calories and not much more. This is heartbreaking, because nutrition has deep healing potential. The opposite is also true: Industrial or processed foods that contain processed sugar, seed oils, additives, preservatives, dyes, pesticides, herbicides, and known carcinogens are associated with a higher risk of chronic disease and are not going to help your child—either in their overall prognosis or in how they feel on a day-to-day basis as their body fights both the cancer and the toxic side effects of treatment.[3]

Sadly, the food served in hospitals is rarely nutritious. It is often fried in oils known to cause cancer.[4] Fruit comes in a plastic cup and swimming in a sugary syrup. Medically recommended formulas and "protein" drinks often contain corn syrup as the first ingredient and sugar as the second. I'm not saying that eating these foods during inpatient treatment will be the straw that breaks the camel's back. What I am saying is: (1) They don't help the body heal. (2) The fact that these are typical protocols is indicative of major blind spots on the part of our medical system. Hospitals employ "dietitians" who are trained using the outdated food pyramid and that a calorie is a calorie. This outdated and harmful approach is still utilized across the country on every pediatric oncology floor.

This is not what I want for your child. Try to identify a nutritionist trained in metabolic and nutritional therapies that use diet to treat cancer. Once you identify an integrative oncology practitioner, they should be able to refer you to an integrative oncology nutritionist.

Other Support

In addition to the integrative medical and nutrition support I recommend incorporating into your child's treatment, it is worth investigating other areas of support as well. For example, cancer care is expensive, and you may need financial support. Start with your hospital's social worker and ask for resources, financial and otherwise. There are many organizations that specifically support integrative therapies either financially or with free education and resources. You can find some of these organizations in appendix D.

Likewise, you may need to find sources of emotional support. Cancer can stir up lots of feelings in the whole family. Do not wait. Get a qualified therapist for all children and a marriage therapist for you and your spouse, if you have one. Finally, find out if your hospital offers physical, occupational, or play therapy. Consider other healing modalities, such as acupuncture, Reiki, and massage therapy (for your child, your other family members, *and* you). Your hospital's child life services program should be able to help identify these and other avenues of support. Don't underestimate the help you might need. Set yourself up for it now, as much as possible.

Legal Issues

One major difference between adult and pediatric oncology care is that an adult has the right to decide what treatment they would like to pursue. Unfortunately, in the United States and many other countries, the law says that a child and their parent(s) do not have that right. While this law exists to protect the child, it can just as easily hurt a child. The problem is that conventional oncology, like most Western medicine, follows recipes or protocols for types of cancer. It is the child, however, that we should be treating—not their cancer. In many situations, because the treatment is not individualized, it fails the patient.

It often happens that a particular chemotherapy or radiation treatment doesn't work for a particular child. Sometimes, even when a child is suffering tremendously with little benefit, doctors might continue to push a treatment. Parents who request to stop the treatment may be denied. I have worked with many families who have successfully refused treatment. I have also worked with many families who were unsuccessful doing so.

There is a vast range in how these situations are handled, and it is often highly subjective. It comes down to your team. It is your child's oncologist who will make the decision to either allow you to stop treatment—or call Child Protective Services if you refuse treatment. This is why it is so important to make sure you trust and have confidence in your child's medical team and choose your child's oncologist carefully. Ask detailed questions during primary and secondary opinions. Pick the right team and get an integrative practitioner on board.

CHAPTER 3

Conduct Additional Testing

A CANCER DIAGNOSIS IS ESTABLISHED THROUGH TESTING. OFTEN, A diagnosis is the result of parents advocating and trying to convince their child's pediatrician that something isn't right—until a blood test or an MRI shows "suspected cancer." In most situations, a definitive diagnosis will be made with a biopsy. As I've mentioned, it's not uncommon for children to be rushed into treatment immediately after initial diagnosis but before confirmation by biopsy, without their parents having all the information they need to make sound decisions. Nor is it uncommon for initial diagnoses to be incorrect. A second opinion, ideally from a different medical institution, is essential.

In this chapter you will learn about testing. I'll cover initial baseline testing, which is essential in establishing health markers *before* treatment begins. Treatment will alter the body immediately, after which it will be too late to conduct this important baseline testing.

This testing will also offer crucial insight into your child's broken "terrain," something I'll cover in more depth in chapter 4. In addition to conventional baseline testing such as complete blood count (CBC) and comprehensive metabolic panel (CMP), I recommend baseline integrative testing, such as tests that assess gut health and epigenetics, and testing for toxins such as glyphosate. It will make sense to repeat many of these tests periodically throughout treatment.

Your metabolic oncology practitioner will be able to guide you in what tests to order, but be aware that these practitioners often have long waiting lists for initial consultation and, while you don't want to rush into treatment, you also don't have time to waste. Therefore, I will provide you with information and recommendations so that you can act on them before your child begins conventional treatment, whether you have identified your metabolic oncology practitioner or not. This chapter will offer an overview of the tests you may want to consider. Appendix A offers details on how to interpret the results of these tests.

You may already know that pediatric anticancer therapy has not advanced much in the last few decades. The good news, however, is that testing has improved dramatically. We are now able to identify cancer earlier and more accurately. Once you learn about the testing that is available, you might be surprised to discover how few tests have been ordered by your child's medical team—tests that could potentially yield insight into your child's health and healing. These tests can help you discover factors that may have contributed to your child's cancer as well as signposts to monitor during and after treatment.

Depending on your child's particular case, most teams will check CBC and CMP monthly, weekly, or even daily (for leukemia during inpatient treatment). It's really on an individual, case-by-case basis, depending on numerous factors, including the type of cancer and the type of results that come back. That said, I can't emphasize enough how valuable it is to conduct baseline testing before treatment begins and monthly thereafter.

Many of my patient's families are surprised to hear that I am just as interested in test results as conventional oncologists are. An integrative metabolic approach to cancer is just as backed by science and evidence as the medical approach is; in fact, I would argue that we test more frequently and thoroughly than conventional oncologists. Dr. Nasha Winters has pioneered the model of "Test, Assess, and Address," which relies on a continual feedback loop of making treatment decisions, monitoring the outcome, and then adapting the treatment in response to how the patient's body responds to the treatment decision. Too often in conventional oncology, patients are put on protocols and, even when the protocols are failing, oncologists continue to push them. Through frequent and thorough testing, we can change course and adjust patient support based on their individual response to therapy. Testing is a powerful tool.

These are the conventional tests I recommend to establish a baseline before conventional treatment starts (and periodically thereafter). I have included summaries of each of these tests, but please consult appendix A for details on how to interpret the results of these tests.

1. Complete blood count (CBC)
2. Comprehensive metabolic panel (CMP)
3. Highly sensitive C-reactive protein (CRP-HS)
4. Erythrocyte sedimentation rate (ESR, or "sed rate")
5. Lactate dehydrogenase (LDH) and isoenzymes
6. Vitamin D3
7. Hemoglobin A1c (HbA1c), insulin, insulin-like growth factor 1 (IGF-1)
8. Ferritin
9. Homocysteine
10. Thyroid
11. Serum copper, zinc, magnesium

Complete Blood Count (CBC)

As its name suggests, the complete blood count (CBC) measures the different types of cells found in the blood—both mature and immature red blood cells and different types of white blood cells such as lymphocytes and neutrophils—as well as platelets (cell fragments) and hemoglobin (a protein that carries oxygen to the cells).

The CBC measures complete count by volume, as cells per liter, grams per deciliter (dL), microliter per cubic milliliter (mL3) or femtoliter (fL). The CBC also measures ratios, such as concentration of hemoglobin and neutrophil to lymphocyte ratios.

The CBC is a common test and will likely be ordered by your child's pediatrician or primary care physician. It is extremely important for blood cancers, naturally, but it can offer valuable information for all cancers. Your child's metabolic oncology practitioner will also be interested in the results of this test but may pay attention to different parts of it.

Comprehensive Metabolic Panel (CMP)

A complete metabolic panel, or CMP, is a blood test that measures fourteen different substances in the blood. It essentially offers a snapshot of the body's chemistry, providing key information about the kidneys, liver, electrolytes, blood sugar, hydration, protein, gut health, and more. The CMP can be especially valuable prior to treatment. Once treatment begins, a CMP should be done at least once a month to assess the impact of treatment on vital organs.

Note that it is not uncommon to see liver markers of AST (aspartate aminotransferase), ALT (alanine transaminase), and total bilirubin elevated during chemotherapy. Creatinine is essential to monitor to be sure the kidneys are not being injured by treatment, as is BUN (blood urea nitrogen) to determine the child's hydration status. A decrease in creatinine, albumin, and total protein will show if malnutrition is an issue. For solid tumors, the CMP is an essential way to monitor how treatment is affecting the child—not necessarily if treatment is working but if it is causing irregularities and toxicities.

The Trifecta Labs (CRP-HS, ESR, LDH)

There are three conventional lab tests, known as the "trifecta labs," that offer tremendous insight into the efficacy of treatment and progress toward healing. A lot of literature exists on each of these markers individually as assessment tools. Dr. Winters pioneered the use of these three labs *together* as a way to conduct monthly monitoring on signs of infection, inflammation, or cancer on the move. All tests—but these in particular—are powerful tools to help the practitioner evaluate the patient and the therapies (conventional or integrative) and evaluate whether a given approach is appropriate for a given patient and situation.

- Highly sensitive C-reactive protein (CRP-HS)
- Erythrocyte sedimentation rate (ESR, or "sed rate")
- Lactate dehydrogenase (LDH) and isoenzymes

C-reactive protein (CRP) is a protein found in the plasma whose concentrations increase when there is inflammation in the body. If elevated, CRP can indicate multiple drug resistance or side effects from treatment. CRP is very important and should be used through standard-of-care treatment and beyond.

The erythrocyte sedimentation rate (ESR, or "sed rate") is useful for determining the level of tissue destruction. This test shows us how sticky our blood is. Elevated sed rate is common in autoimmune disease.

Lactate dehydrogenase (LDH) is an enzyme of the anaerobic metabolic pathway. When it increases, it can indicate tissue damage. It also suggests if the body's terrain is "welcoming" to cancer; it is a tumor marker for lymphoma and leukemia. For solid tumors it helps us evaluate the tumor microenvironment and tells us the rate of cell division. It can also indicate damage to organs such as the liver, lungs, heart, or kidneys. For more specifics, ask your child's metabolic oncology practitioner to order an LDH isoenzyme.

Do note, however, that LDH can often be elevated in kids when they are going through a growth spurt. This would typically show as elevated isoenzymes LDH 1 and LDH 2. For this reason, LDH is less reliable as an inflammatory marker for children than it is for adults.

Ferritin

Serum ferritin, the protein that stores iron in your blood, is the body's main iron storage site. Many pediatric cancer patients end up with iron overload from blood transfusions. The initial treatment for this is therapeutic phlebotomy—weekly bloodletting—to decrease the serum ferritin. If serum ferritin is over 1,000 nanograms per milliliter, an MRI should be ordered to assess iron deposits in organs such as the liver and heart. If serum ferritin is high, your metabolic oncology practitioner should investigate the cause with a total serum iron test, and if serum ferritin is low, evaluate with a total iron-binding capacity test (TIBC).

Homocysteine

Homocysteine is an amino acid. Vitamin B12, B6, and folate break it down to create other chemicals your body needs. Levels of homocysteine are typically low because available vitamin B12, B6, and folate get used up so quickly, so high homocysteine levels indicate vitamin B12, B6, and folate deficiencies or that the process of breaking down homocysteine isn't functioning properly. High homocysteine levels can also be due to genetic or epigenetic factors, such as the MTHFR SNP, or poor gut absorption.

An MTHFR mutation, which affects our ability to methylate, is common in pediatric cancer patients. Methylation has many functions. One of them is to aid in the breakdown of many chemo drugs; another is to aid in the suppression of tumor formation. Elevated homocysteine might prompt a practitioner to test for epigenetic mutation of MTHFR and support accordingly. Supplementing methylated vitamin B can lower homocysteine.

Thyroid

It is important to conduct baseline thyroid testing on all pediatric cancer patients because chemotherapy and, especially, radiation near the thyroid can result in thyroid disease down the line. Endocrine problems are a common late effect of many pediatric cancer survivors. Once you have a baseline, I suggest checking the thyroid every six to twelve months to see how it is being affected by treatment. There also are some children who go into treatment with a poorly functioning thyroid; it is important to catch this in advance so that the appropriate medications can be started. Healthy thyroid function is necessary for proper treatment response and healing.

Vitamin D3

Multiple clinical studies suggest that vitamin D3 deficiency increases the risk of developing cancer and is associated with overall lower rates of survival.[1] Vitamin D3 has been shown to help reverse drug resistance in cancer cells, improve outcomes in pediatric cancer, including ALL.[2] The anticancer effects of vitamin D may be due to its role in controlling cell growth, differentiation, apoptosis, and angiogenesis. Vitamin D may also inhibit processes that stimulate tumor progression. Overall, vitamin D appears to have an association with reduced cancer risk, but more research is needed to establish its definitive preventative and therapeutic roles.

It is important for cancer patients and survivors to maintain levels of vitamin D over 50 nanomoles per liter. Low vitamin D can lead to osteoporosis, depression, and immune system dysregulation. Maintaining adequate vitamin D is a simple and safe way to reduce cancer incidence and improve cancer prognosis and outcomes in all patients.

Hemoglobin A1c (HbA1c), Insulin, Insulin-Like Growth Factor-1 (IGF-1)

Here's the bad news: There is a clear correlation between diabetes and cancer.[3] Here's the worse news: Only 7 percent of US adults are metabolically healthy, and the number of children under the age of twenty living with type 2 diabetes grew by 95 percent between 2010 and 2017.[4] Unfortunately, it is not uncommon for me to see children at my clinic who have been diagnosed with cancer and are also prediabetic or diabetic. Their parents often don't even know; it is not standard to check the relevant labs on kids unless they have symptoms.

There are several relevant lab tests for metabolic health. Fasting insulin should ideally be under 5; some practitioners even say 3. Fasting glucose (from a CMP) should be under 90. Hemoglobin A1c (HbA1c) should be 5.3 or less.

The reference ranges given on your child's lab results are not an indication of health; disregard them because prediabetic markers are referred to as normal in conventional medicine. Instead, use the reference ranges I have given here.

Insulin-like growth factor 1 (IGF-1) is a hormone that helps regulate growth hormone. IGF-I serum level is an important indicator of risk for the most prevalent forms of childhood cancer and is known to promote cancer development by inhibiting apoptosis and stimulating cell proliferation.[5] Children with cancer typically have significantly higher levels of IGF-1 than their healthy peers do, but note that IGF-1 can also be elevated from stress or lack of sleep. Depressed levels can indicate growth deficiency, most commonly due to cancer treatment.

In integrative medicine, we use IGF differently. It is not an uncommon late effect for children who went through cancer treatment to have growth hormone deficiency; this is also tracked by checking IGF-1.[6]

Magnesium, Zinc, and Copper

Magnesium is essential to health. It reduces constipation, aids in muscle relaxation, and helps reduce anxiety—all of which can be issues when living with cancer. Magnesium is also easy to supplement; it can be used generally or in specific situations such as to prevent cisplatin-induced kidney injury.[7] Chemotherapy and immunotherapies can impact magnesium levels. During these treatments, it may make sense to check magnesium monthly.

Zinc is a trace mineral, but one that is essential for approximately one hundred different enzymes to carry out essential functions. It is essential to immune system and metabolic function and plays a role in cell growth, DNA production, wound healing, and building proteins. It is found in foods such as beef, poultry, and pork, and can also be given as a supplement. Supplementing with zinc can help reduce the severity of oropharyngeal mucositis in children undergoing certain chemotherapies.[8] It can be helpful to have a baseline zinc level, but it's only necessary to retest if you're supplementing for a long time.

Copper helps your body make red blood cells and collagen. It can reduce free radicals and helps keep your nerve cells and immune system stay healthy. However, it also plays a role in cancer cell growth and proliferation.[9] It can be valuable to check copper levels at least once as part of an initial lab panel. It should also be noted that zinc and copper have an indirect relationship: Zinc reduces the amount of copper your body can absorb. I check zinc and copper together to be sure that one is not affecting the other.

Imaging

There are many ways to understand what's going on inside the body. For children with solid tumors, in particular, imaging will also be a part of their testing. While incredibly useful, unfortunately, imaging carries its own health risks. It is important to understand the kind of imaging your child's oncologist is recommending as well as the frequency with which it is being used. CT scans and X-rays use ionized radiation, which can damage DNA and increase the risk of—you guessed it—cancer. The American College of Radiology recommends limiting your lifetime diagnostic radiation exposure to 100 mSv, or approximately twenty-five CT scans.

Gadolinium is a chemical element used as a contrast agent in both MRIs and CT scans and is known to be harmful to the kidneys.[10] In addition to kidney damage or acute renal failure, there have been cases of gadolinium accumulation in other tissue, such as the bones and brain, even when no renal impairment is present, and the FDA is currently evaluating the risk of brain deposits with repeated use of gadolinium-based contrast agents for MRIs.[11] If your child is going to have imaging contrast administered, make sure they are well hydrated and request that they be given the maximum amount of IV normal saline per body weight to help flush the kidneys afterward. Investigate options for alternative ways to monitor your child's disease process and ask your team about safer spacing of imaging procedures or eliminating contrast altogether.

For MRI/CT radiation *and* contrast mitigation, I recommend:

- Stopping mistletoe at least seventy-two hours, or up to two weeks, prior
- Stopping IV vitamin C at least forty-eight hours prior
- No strenuous exercise twenty-four hours prior
- A high-protein, low-carbohydrate diet, twenty-four hours prior
- No food or drink, other than water, six hours prior
- Vitamin D3: 2,000 to 20,000 IU, depending on age and weight, day of the scan
- Fish oil: 500 milligrams to 4 grams, depending on age and weight, day of the scan

- Probiotic: three times, day of the scan
- Liposomal glutathione: one or two pumps, day of the scan
- Melatonin: 50 to 200 milligrams, depending on age and weight, day of the scan

Other antioxidant protectants at your discretion include green tea extract, vitamin E, NAC, vitamin A, pomegranate, milk thistle, and turmeric.

In addition to common imaging technologies—ultrasound, X-ray, CT scan, PET scan, MRI—there is now emerging technology for improved, lower risk imaging. Some of the pros and cons of each are described below.

Ultrasound. An ultrasound uses sound waves to create a picture of organs, tissue, and other structures in the body. Because ultrasound does not use radiation, it is considered the safest of the imaging technologies. However, it is not the most accurate way of seeing solid tumors and therefore is not used very often. You might wish to speak to your child's oncology team about using ultrasound as an alternative to radiation-based imaging technologies.

X-ray. X-rays are a type of radiation called electromagnetic waves. The images they produce show parts of the body in shades of black and white. A single chest X-ray exposes the patient to about 0.1 mSv, which is far less than a CT scan, so you may wish to ask your child's oncology team about using X-rays instead of CT scans, if and when possible.

Computed tomography (CT) scan. A CT scan uses a series of X-rays and a computer to produce a single 3D image of soft tissue and bones. It is a useful diagnostic tool, but radiation exposure from a single CT scan can range between 7 and 20 mSv, depending on the size of the area being scanned (for example, the entire body or just part of the body). That is a lot of radiation exposure, especially for a child, and should therefore be limited to clinical and diagnostic necessity.

Positron emission tomography (PET) scan. A PET scan is an imaging test that uses radioactive substances known as radiotracers. To find malignant tumors, a small amount of radioactive glucose (sugar) is injected into a vein and then the PET scanner is applied to detect the distribution of the sugar in the tumor and in the body. (Cancer loves sugar, so the sugar goes right to the malignant cancer cells.) PET scans have an approximate radiation exposure of 8 mSv.

Magnetic resonance imaging (MRI). Unlike X-ray, CT, and PET scans, MRIs do not use ionizing radiation. Instead, they use strong magnetic field and radio waves to take pictures. However, MRIs do come with their own risks. The contrast agent gadolinium is used, and the MRI's magnetic field is exceptionally strong. This can result in kidney injury as well as deposits left in the brain and bone referred to as gadolinium deposition disease.

Prenuvo scan. There are emerging alternative imaging technologies, such as the Prenuvo scan. This is a whole-body, radiation-free MRI. As this book goes to press, there are six locations in the United States where the Prenuvo scan is offered and ten more coming soon. Unfortunately, they are not yet an option for children.

––––––––

In the remainder of this chapter, I'll cover additional testing that you may want to explore with your child's metabolic oncology practitioner. There are endless options for this type of testing, so I recommend that you work with your child's metabolic oncology practitioner to identify what you want to target, gather the clinician's recommendations, and ask them to help you interpret the results. While some of these tests can be ordered by you without going through a practitioner, they can be hard to interpret without experience reading the results.

I've included further details on these tests in appendix A, including approximate cost when available (at the time of this writing) and my recommendations for companies to use. Your child's metabolic oncology practitioner will likely have recommendations as well. The value of some of these tests will become more clear in chapter 4, which goes into detail on how to assess your child's terrain.

All that said, don't discount other methods of data collection. Some, such as elimination diets, are free or low cost, and infinitely valuable.

Genetic and Epigenetic Testing

After your child has been diagnosed, ask your child's oncology team if there is any genetic testing that is available for the type of cancer your child has. Depending on the type of cancer your child has, genetic testing might reveal information that will help your child's oncologist make treatment decisions. For example, for acute myeloid leukemia, genetic testing can reveal the relative risk of treatment approaches such as chemo alone versus chemo and bone marrow transplant. For solid tumors it helps identify particular treatments that may be targeted toward just that genetic mutation.

In addition to genetic testing that may be recommended by your child's conventional oncology team, integrative care offers options for epigenetic testing. An epigenetic test provides insight into your child's unique epigenetic profile, including information on methylation, hormones, inflammation, toxin sensitivity, nutrition, and more. The best-case scenario is that it will offer insight into why your child was vulnerable to cancer in the first place, as well as what type of diet and supplements will support your child during and following treatment. It can help inform decisions regarding chemotherapy, as well as offer clues on what therapies might support detoxification from chemotherapy. See appendix A for recommendations.

Microbiome Testing

The human microbiome is a collection of mostly beneficial bacteria and other microorganisms that play crucial roles in our physiological functioning. Sadly, anticancer therapies kill many of these beneficial bacteria, disrupt the microbial balance, and destroy the gut's protective lining, which is crucial to nutrient absorption and to blocking pathogens and inflammatory molecules from leaking into the blood stream and circulating throughout the body. Chemotherapy, radiation, immunotherapies, antibiotics, steroids, and antipyretics contribute to ruining the ability of our intestines to absorb.

Every child with cancer should have their microbiome tested at some point, ideally before starting treatment. Prior to treatment, the state of the microbiome can offer insight into whether dysbiosis may have contributed to the development of their cancer (see chapter 4). After treatment, it can be used to assess treatment damage to the gut and inform gut-healing protocols. Appendix A contains details on microbiome testing that you can order and interpret with the help of your child's metabolic oncology practitioner.

Because the microbiome is so essential to health and healing, I devote an entire chapter to it (see chapter 11).

Food Sensitivity

Although food sensitivity tests are commonly ordered in functional medicine, the best food sensitivity test is the elimination diet, a methodical process of eliminating certain foods from the diet for a period of time and then slowly reincorporating them, one at a time, while carefully assessing and recording the body's response. I know a quick test seems so much easier than the time and effort involved in an elimination diet, but food sensitivity tests are often inaccurate. An elimination diet really is your best bet, in most cases.

There are many variations of the elimination diet, customized for the patient. A good, general protocol to begin is to eliminate all potentially triggering foods—including gluten (or all grains), dairy, nuts, nightshades, processed sugars, artificial colors, and refined seed oils—for at least three weeks. Choose one group and slowly add it back to your child's diet for three to four days. Observe your child's reaction to it. Make gluten the final food type you add back in, since it sometimes needs to be eliminated for as long as three months in order to feel the benefit. The Institute for Functional Medicine has published a comprehensive elimination diet guide for reference.[12]

Toxicity Testing

Since environmental toxins are hugely implicated in pediatric cancers and pollutants are now so ubiquitous, I like to conduct toxicity testing on all pediatric cancer patients, even if they don't score high on the toxicity terrain questionnaire (see chapter 4). I also tend to order toxicity tests for patients who have certain single nucleotide polymorphisms (SNPs) on their Nutrition Genome test (see appendix A); this shows me they either are a sponge for certain toxins or have hiccups in their liver pathways that reduce detoxification capacity. Most of my pediatric cancer patients have water-soluble (glyphosate) and fat-soluble toxins in their body. Depending on the patient's exposure, I develop a detoxification plan.

I think it is important to test for glyphosate, in particular, since the link between glyphosate exposure and cancer, especially blood cancers, is mounting. Glyphosate is water-soluble and the urine test is very accurate, which means that if the test is high, your child is *currently* being exposed. Thankfully, detox through elimination, such as sweating, is also

easier. I discuss how to detox from glyphosate in chapter 10. Unfortunately, no one is "glyphosate-free" anymore. I have never seen a single
negative glyphosate test, so that's not what I'm looking for. Some children's exposure is as much as 800 percent higher than normal. With the
right detoxification plan I have seen these high levels of glyphosate clear
in many of my patients.

Heavy Metal Testing

Practically speaking, heavy metal toxicity is less of an issue in childhood cancer. That is to say, in my experience, it doesn't turn up very often in testing.
I do not routinely order heavy metal toxicity testing for my patients unless I
have a reason to suspect exposure at higher levels than typical. (For example,
if a family lives near a factory or other highly polluted area.)

That said, heavy metal toxicity, when it does happen, can be devastating,
and some families would simply like to know if they have been exposed.
There are a few different ways to get a heavy metal test, including a provoked
chelation test, which I do not recommend for children. (Provoked means
that the patient is administered a heavy metal chelator, which is a medicine
that binds heavy metals, prior to the test and then gives a urine sample.)
Chelation, when not done correctly, can be dangerous. For children, it is safer
to use a urine test without the chelator.

Hormone Testing

Hormone testing is also less applicable to children than adults. Overall, children are less likely to suffer from hormonally driven cancers because they
don't tend to have an excess of sex hormones prior to puberty. However, it
is not unheard of, and I worry that hormonally driven cancers in children
may be becoming more common with increased exposure to xenoestrogens,
which are estrogen-mimicking compounds people are exposed to through
food, toiletries, and household products.

When I conduct hormone testing, it is most commonly for preteens and
teens who have undergone a bone marrow transplant prior to puberty or
first menses and who may be taking bioidentical hormones to stimulate
puberty. Hormone blood testing is not very accurate; I prefer to use urine
testing to identify the balance of hormones and keep an eye out for estrogen
dominance, or too much estrogen in the body.

Immune System Testing

There is a new test that allows for screening of the immune system. This is an excellent test for patients using immune-system-modulating therapies including mistletoe or patients post bone marrow transplant.

Circulating Tumor Cell Testing

Finally, circulating tumor cell (CTC) testing provides a blood work biomarker for early cancer detection, progression, or treatment effectiveness.[13] The biggest issue with CTC testing is the validity of the testing company. There are a few companies out there that charge patients lots of money but do not provide accurate information. (Many of these tests are, however, covered by insurance.) I am choosing not to list any companies in the book, as this is an ever-changing arena. I recommend you speak with your child's metabolic oncology practitioner.

You've now conducted baseline testing, which offers you a lot of information. These lab tests can help you understand what factors may have contributed to your child's illness. For example, an elevated fasting glucose or fasting insulin might suggest that blood sugar dysregulation may have contributed to the development of cancer.

Of course, not every abnormal lab test result points to the cause of cancer. But it is a fact that environmental factors can influence the development of cancer. I refer to these factors as the "terrain." In the next chapter I will explore the different lenses through which one can understand how a child becomes vulnerable to cancer and what you, as the parent, can do about it.

CHAPTER 4

Assess the Terrain

IN THEIR GROUNDBREAKING BOOK, *THE METABOLIC APPROACH TO CANCER*, Dr. Nasha Winters and Jess Higgins Kelley describe ten factors that have an impact on the development of cancer and our ability to overcome it.[1] These ten factors, which they've termed "The Terrain Ten" are:

The Terrain Ten™
1. Genetic, epigenetic, and nutrigenomic modifications
2. Blood sugar balance
3. Toxic burden management
4. Repopulating and balancing the microbiome
5. Immune system maximization
6. Modulating inflammation and oxidative stress
7. Enhancing blood circulation while inhibiting angiogenesis and metastasis
8. Establishing hormone balance
9. Recalibrating stress levels and biorhythms
10. Enhancing mental and emotional well-being

In this chapter, I have adapted the questionnaire developed by Winters and Kelley to pediatric patients, simplifying it to combine stress and emotional health, as well as omitting blood circulation (because although circulatory issues can contribute to the development of cancer in children, this factor is far more applicable to adults).

In order to gather some additional baseline data that will inform your integrative care strategies, answer each of these eight sets of questions for your child. For every yes, note a "1" next to the question, then add up each category. The categories with the three highest scores are where I recommend you begin to focus your attention in terms of integrative care and support for your child.

Genetics and Epigenetics

1. Does the child have a family history of cancer?
2. Has the child tested positive for any type of gene mutation?
3. Were the child's parents exposed to large amounts of stress or environmental toxins?
4. Did the child's mother smoke, drink alcohol, or take any drugs or medications while pregnant or planning to get pregnant?
5. Is the child homozygous or heterozygous for MTHFR?
6. Was there any trauma or major stress in the child's grandparents' lives?
7. Is the child on any pharmaceutical medications, including over-the-counter medications?
8. Has the child experienced any kind of trauma?

Blood Sugar Balance

1. Does the child have a sweet tooth?
2. Does the child get hungry before bed, in the middle of the night, or very early in the day?
3. Does the child get hangry?
4. Are sweet foods the child's comfort / craving food?
5. Is the child overweight?
6. Does the child crave sugar after a meal or feel tired after eating?
7. Does anyone in the child's family have metabolic syndrome, diabetes, PCOS, pancreatitis, or insulin issues?
8. Does the child consume more than 25 grams of sugar per day?

Toxic Burden

1. Has the child lived, or does the child currently live, near a golf course, airport, toxic waste site, factory, military base, or agricultural area like a farm?
2. Has the child been or is the child currently exposed to a microwave, cell phone, laptop computer, Fitbit-like product, or baby monitor for more than three hours per day?
3. Does the child have sensitivities to odors like perfumes or diesel fuel?
4. Does the child live in a place where pesticides or herbicides are sprayed in or around the home (including for bugs or mosquitos) or on pets (including tick guards)?

5. Is the child exposed to nonorganic toiletries or cleaning products like body wash or laundry detergent? Does the child have a nonorganic mattress, flame-retardant clothing, or not launder new clothes before wearing them?
6. Is the child exposed to nonstick cookware or plastic food containers?
7. Does the child have a history of second- or third-hand cigarette smoke?
8. Does the child have mercury fillings or heavy metal exposure?

Microbiome

1. Was the child born via cesarean delivery?
2. Was the child fed infant formula before the age of one?
3. Did the child get antibiotics under the age of three or multiple courses of antibiotics under the age of twelve?
4. Does the child have digestive symptoms like constipation, diarrhea, or bloating?
5. Does the child eat nonorganic meat or dairy?
6. Has the child had multiple doses of acetaminophen or ibuprofen?
7. Does the child eat foods made from processed, nonorganic grains, such as bread and pasta?
8. Does the child use hand sanitizer or antimicrobial soap?

Immune Function

1. Has the child been administered acetaminophen or ibuprofen to suppress a fever?
2. Has the child been diagnosed with an autoimmune disease or does the child have a family history of autoimmune disease?
3. Is the child's vitamin D3 low?
4. Is the child always sick?
5. Does the child have any allergies?
6. Does the child have gluten intolerance?
7. Has the child been vaccinated?
8. Has the child ever been administered steroids?

Inflammation

1. Does the child have a history of eczema, acne, flushing, or rashes?
2. Does the child have joint pain?

3. Does the child have inflammatory bowel disease (ulcerative colitis or Crohn's disease)?
4. Does the child eat fried food or fast food?
5. Does the child have any food allergies or reflux?
6. Is the child administered NSAIDs such as ibuprofen?
7. Does the child not eat vegetables daily?
8. Is the child overweight?

Hormones

1. Has the child taken birth control pills, bioidentical or standard hormone replacement therapy, or hormone blockade therapies?
2. Did the child have early puberty before age ten or early menses?
3. Does the child drink out of plastic bottles or have exposure to products containing parabens?
4. Does the child eat nonorganic animal protein more than once per month?
5. Has the child been diagnosed with a thyroid disorder?
6. Has the child taken steroids in the past or used a steroid inhaler?
7. Has the child been diagnosed with adrenal fatigue?
8. Does the child have weight fluctuations or ever follow a low-fat diet?

Stress and Emotional Health

1. Did a stressful event precede the cancer diagnosis (for example, death, move, divorce)?
2. Does the child crave salt?
3. Does the child sleep fewer than eight hours per night? (Or not nap if they're under four years old?)
4. Does the child have screen time after 5 p.m.?
5. Does the child experience mood swings or unstable emotions?
6. Does the child spend less than fifteen minutes outside daily?
7. Has the child been diagnosed with a mental disorder (such as anxiety, depression, or ADD/ADHD)?
8. Does the child feel high levels of stress every day?

Once you calculate your child's score, you will have some additional information on where to focus your energies. That information can run the gamut between somewhat suggestive of what may have contributed to your child's cancer and a smoking gun. For example, in Zuza's case, she scored high in the toxic burden category, especially because we were living behind a cornfield at the time of her diagnosis. This prompted us to test her glyphosate exposure. The results were disturbing, but they also gave us crucial understanding in how to support her through cancer treatment.

As you may know, glyphosate is the active ingredient in the herbicide Roundup, which appeared on the market in 1974. Since then, glyphosate usage boomed in the United States. Glyphosate has been linked to many cancers, including lymphoma and leukemia. A 2016 study found it in 93 percent of urine samples.[2] According to the National Cancer Institute, the rate of pediatric cancer has increased 27 percent since 1975, one year after glyphosate was brought to market, and there is a mountain of evidence linking childhood cancer and exposure to agricultural chemicals.[3]

A recent study found that exposure to certain pesticides during pregnancy due to residential proximity to agricultural applications may increase the risk of childhood ALL and AML.[4] A 2021 study showed that insecticides and herbicides are both associated with higher risk of childhood leukemia.[5] A 2020 Danish study showed that mothers who lived within ½ kilometer of crops increased their risk of having children with childhood leukemia.[6] Another 2021 study showed a threefold increase in risk for ALL was observed among children in very close proximity (less than 75 meters) to outdoor plant nurseries.[7] In 2019, researchers at University of Washington concluded that using glyphosate increases the risk of non-Hodgkin lymphoma by 41 percent.[8]

All of this is to say that the results of this questionnaire might point to additional testing you may wish to invest in, something I'll cover in greater detail in chapter 5. This questionnaire should be considered a starting point—a place to begin. As such, even if your child scored low in certain categories, I still recommend you read all the summaries and give some attention to how each terrain factor might be impacting your child's cancer, health, and potential recovery.

As you do this, it is important not to get into the self-blame game. I say this because I know how our parental minds work: We hold ourselves responsible for everything. If, like Zuza, your child has high levels of toxic exposure because you live next to a farm field, or if they have a compromised microbiome because they were born by cesarean, it may be very hard not to beat yourself up over it. But there is no blame here. This is not your fault. The true failure rests with the companies who produce these products, the regulatory agencies that fail to protect the public from them, and the lawmakers who look the other way—or even benefit from these practices. And—this is important—blaming yourself or beating yourself up will not help your child. In the coming weeks, months, and years, you are going to be facing situations that no parent and no child should ever have to experience. You are going to need to make difficult decisions about your child's care and there will be a million opportunities to doubt, second-guess, or blame yourself. Do not indulge in this. I repeat: The self-blame game will not help your child. Your child needs you to be empowered and productive.

That said—and this is a crucial nuance—you need to investigate, you need to be aware, and you need to ask yourself difficult questions. You need to look at your lifestyle, your family's nutrition, where you live, and the products in your home and ask yourself some difficult questions about what may have contributed to—or possibly even caused—your child's cancer.

Your child's oncologist will probably tell you that there is nothing you did to cause this diagnosis. They are trying to be compassionate, and they may even believe that cancer is just genetic bad luck. Of course, there is an element of genetics. But we also know that up to 95 percent of cancers are caused by environmental toxins.[9] There are many, many known carcinogens that your child has almost certainly been exposed to—that we are all exposed to—because, sadly, human health—including the health and lives of children—has too often taken a back seat to corporate profits, and the US regulatory agencies have not done a good job of protecting the health of American children. This is not your fault. This is something for you to be aware of. As your child's advocate, it is your responsibility to evaluate what may have contributed to your child's cancer. Conventional oncology skips this step. I do not.

In the next chapter, I'll go into more detail about how you might interpret the results of this terrain questionnaire, with more information on each of the categories, before delving into the important role of nutrition in chapter 6.

CHAPTER 5

Address the Terrain

IN THE PREVIOUS CHAPTER, I INTRODUCED YOU TO THE CONCEPT OF terrain, as developed by Dr. Nasha Winters and Jess Higgins Kelley in their book *The Metabolic Approach to Cancer*, and offered you a simple tool, adapted from Winters and Kelley's own assessment. The goal of that tool is to give you a framework to begin to understand how your child's terrain may be compromised, how that situation may have contributed to their cancer, and areas you may want to focus on in terms of integrative support for their health and healing.

In this chapter, I'll dive a little deeper into each of the terrain areas and offer you some tools and information to pursue for each category. Then, I'll look at additional testing, both conventional and integrative, that you may wish to pursue (and, in appendix A, information on how to interpret the results) before turning attention to the important subject of nutrition. (Indeed, regardless of which aspect of your child's terrain is most compromised, in the metabolic approach, nutrition is always the lynchpin of healing.)

As I mentioned at the end of chapter 4, even if your child did not score high on a given terrain category, I recommend reading through the summaries anyway. You never know when new information or developments in your child's health or disease progression might bring one of these other categories to the forefront of your attention. And, as you have likely perceived, none of these terrain categories exists in a silo. At the end of the day, I am always looking at the whole child and the big picture.

Genetics and Epigenetics

While genetics can influence disease processes, they do not dictate these processes, as many have been led to believe. In fact, by some estimates, genetics cause only 5 to 10 percent of cancers.[1] This means that diet, exercise, toxic exposure, anxiety and stress, food allergens, infections, and other lifestyle factors play a much larger role than is typically acknowledged by conventional oncology. This also means you have more power to help your child than you may think.

Epigenetics refers to changes in cell function that don't involve changes to DNA. Epigenetics are not fixed in the same way the DNA sequence is. Think of epigenetics as the genome's light switch, flipping cell responses and functions on and off depending on countless environmental factors. Genetic variations can be latent, becoming harmful under certain conditions. These changes can cause people to be at higher risk for cancer after exposure to certain environmental agents, which may help explain why certain kids respond well to certain chemotherapy drugs and other interventions and others do not.

The most common type of genetic variation is a single nucleotide polymorphism (SNP), defined as a single base change in a DNA sequence. SNPs can cause harmful, harmless, or latent effects. SNPs may cause subtle changes in a group of genes that under normal conditions stay "switched off," but that "switch on," for example, when your child is exposed to a certain carcinogen. SNPs also explain why some patients respond well to a drug treatment whereas others may experience organ failure from the same treatment. Many proteins interact with the drug, affecting the transportation of it throughout the body, as well as absorption and excretion. If your child has SNPs in any of these processes, it may alter the effectiveness and toxicity of a particular drug.

MTHFR SNP

The MTHFR SNP is of particular interest with respect to childhood cancer because kids with this mutation have up to a 70 percent reduction of normal MTHFR enzyme activity compared to those who do not. This results in poor methylation, a process crucial for immune, neurological, and detoxification systems. The Nutrition Genome test (see appendix A) can help you identify if your child has an MTHFR mutation.

We can improve methylation with folate-rich foods and methylated B vitamins. Folate can be found in spinach, bok choy, romaine lettuce, asparagus, goose and duck liver, mustard and turnip greens, beets, and Brussels sprouts. Folate deficiency can result in fatigue, anemia, thyroid problems, and possibly anxiety. (Folic acid is added to grains but individuals with the MTHFR SNP can't use folic acid; they need methylated folate for adequate absorption.) Folate level can be checked through standard conventional blood work.

Folate is particularly relevant to patients with ALL because the antifolate chemotherapy drug methotrexate is often used in ALL treatment. It acts by preventing cells from making and repairing DNA. It also influences several other stops in the folate pathway, causing cellular folate depletion and inhibition of MTHFR synthesis. In fact, studies show an association between MTHFR SNPs and methotrexate toxicity risk.[2] This is a good example of the impact of a genetic variant on drug response. The reason patients with the MTHFR gene mutation suffer more with severe side effects of antifolate chemotherapy is because their bodies lack the adequate folate necessary to produce nucleotides, which are a key component of DNA repair. This may warrant consideration in terms of treatment.

While MTHFR is common in pediatric cancer patients, other SNPs have also been identified with certain pediatric cancers and their prognosis. For example, Ewing sarcoma has three SNPs—ABCC6, ABCB1, and CYP2C8—that can be useful as prognostic markers.[3] SNPs in the MAPK signaling pathway are associated with ALL risk and should be used as novel markers for ALL susceptibility.[4] SNPs can also help identify chemotherapy drugs that may be more or less effective in your child's treatment.[5]

PON1 SNP

Likewise, the PON1 gene helps detoxify organophosphate pesticides. Many of my pediatric cancer patients have a mutation in this gene, which reduces detoxification capacity. Individuals with this mutation are at an 82 percent higher risk of organophosphate toxicity compared to people without it; if the patient is Caucasian, the risk of toxicity jumps up by 148 percent. Asians are unaffected by this mutation.[6]

What can you do if you know your child has the PON1 SNP? The flavonol quercetin, which is found in foods such as onions, berries, grapes, cherries, broccoli, and citrus, as well as in supplement form, has been shown to increase PON1 by as much as 200 percent. Other foods that can reduce oxidants from inhibiting PON1 include extra virgin olive oil, green tea, dates (Hawaiian variety), pomegranate juice, fish oil, mustard, and wasabi.

––––––––––

There are many other genetic mutations, specifically in the liver pathway and associated with glutathione production, that can contribute to your child's inability to detoxify. Therefore, I can't stress enough the importance of using the Nutrition Genome test (see appendix A) to help individualize your child's healing plan. It provides one hundred clinically relevant genes in eight different targeted areas of digestion, energy, hormones, stress, inflammation, DNA repair, and detoxification. Your integrative practitioner should be able to help identify the pieces of the puzzle that contributed most to your child's cancer.

What can you do? In addition to having your child tested through Nutrition Genome, ask your oncology team if there are any SNPs known to affect your child's cancer or treatment. Do some research yourself: Search your child's cancer diagnosis or chemotherapy protocol and the word SNP. Bring this information to your team to discuss how your child's treatment protocol can be adjusted based on this information. Knowing your child's epigenetics gives you insight into better ways to approach conventional treatment and clues as to what may have contributed to your child's cancer.

Blood Sugar Balance

In 2010, researchers at Harvard Medical School reported that up to 80 percent of cancers are driven by the effects of glucose and insulin and that chronically elevated blood sugar contributes to the progression and recurrence of cancer.[7] It should be of huge concern to everyone, then, that the average American child consumes fifty-three pounds of sugar per year.[8] Cancer cells love sugar. If a child's high sugar consumption doesn't lead to a cancer diagnosis directly, it undoubtedly creates a hospitable environment for cancer cells.

Sugar has infiltrated the human diet, especially the standard American diet, to such an extent that you must truly go out of your way to eliminate it. A bowl of cereal has approximately twelve grams of sugar. Children under the age of eight should consume no more than twelve grams of added sugar *per day*. This is less than three teaspoons.

Is all sugar bad? It depends. It's essential to eliminate high-fructose corn syrup and refined white sugar. Naturally occurring sugars like those in fruit or honey are less harmful. However, these sugars still cause blood sugars to rise and should be restricted during cancer treatment.

Hyperglycemia is a neglected factor during cancer progression in conventional oncology. We have long known that there is a higher incidence of cancer in people with type 2 diabetes, and studies are now showing this is due to hyperglycemia. Hyperglycemia is associated with metastasis and may contribute to cancer cells becoming stronger, more resistant to chemotherapy, and more resistant to cell death in primary lesions.[9] Retrospective studies show that hyperglycemic serum levels during radiation therapy impact patient survival and progression patterns in primary glioblastoma. Studies indicate that the diabetes drug metformin can improve the efficacy of radiotherapy in patients with cancer and diabetes.

But it is not only people with diabetes who need to be concerned about sugar and cancer. According to the Centers for Disease Control and Prevention, one out of three Americans have prediabetes and 84 percent of them don't know it.[10] One in four children has prediabetes. If these children have cancer, they will not have an optimal response to radiation therapy. It is ideal to be in ketosis during radiation therapy (more on this in chapter 6).

Multiple studies show that short-term fasting around chemotherapy not only reduced chemotherapy side effects and toxicities but helped with long-term remission. One study in adults compared breast cancer patients who resumed a regular diet after treatment versus a group that ate a fasting-mimicking diet (FMD) around treatment. The FMD group had a better radiological response and were able to omit the need for dexamethasone (steroids). Even more exciting is that 90 to 100 percent of tumor cell loss, as well as reduced DNA damage in healthy cells and reduced DNA damage in healthy cells, is more likely to occur in patients using an FMD.[11]

If you decided to change only one thing about your child's diet during anticancer treatment, I recommend drastically reducing all sugar and eliminating refined sugar. It has no place in your child's diet during treatment. (If eliminating even natural sweeteners seems like a bridge too far, see chapter 6 for information on alternatives to refined white sugar, such as organic stevia and monk fruit.)

Toxic Burden

More than 200 chemicals can be found in newborn umbilical cord blood.[12] Children have increased susceptibility to carcinogens because they are smaller than adults and their immune system and detoxification pathways are still developing.[13] Chemicals are routinely incorporated into children's products with no preliminary cancer testing. By age two, children have been exposed to most carcinogens that may have contributed to their diagnosis.

Common Carcinogens

- Arsenic
- Benzene
- Cadmium
- Chromium
- Coal tar
- Ethylene oxide
- Formaldehyde
- Mercury
- Methylene glycol
- Mineral oils
- Parabens
- Phenacetin
- Triclosan

Even a breast-fed baby will routinely breathe carcinogens or absorb them through their skin.

Sadly, carcinogens are everywhere: car seats, baby mattresses, clothes, toiletries, cleaning supplies, furniture, food, medication. For example, in 2021, Johnson & Johnson recalled four Neutrogena sunscreen products and one Aveeno product after internal testing detected benzene, a carcinogen. Seventy-eight other batches of sunscreen products were also found to contain benzene.[14] Even worse, Johnson & Johnson was aware for at least fifty years that their baby powder was contaminated with asbestos.[15] Thousands of people developed mesothelioma and ovarian cancer, both linked to asbestos exposure, through baby powder.

Humans ingest carcinogens every day through the food we eat and the water we drink. However, this is an area where you can exert a lot of control by feeding your child real, organic food. A recent study tested the pesticide levels of kids' urine before and after changing to an all-organic food diet and concluded that "an organic diet was associated with significant reductions in urinary excretion of several pesticide metabolites and parent compounds."[16] Each year the Environmental Working Group (EWG) issues a "Dirty Dozen" list of the twelve most heavily contaminated fruits and vegetables; see "The EWG's Dirty Dozen (2023)" on page 60.

Many medications also have been linked to cancer, including those involved in *treating* cancer, such as MiraLAX, acetaminophen, ibuprofen, and proton-pump inhibitors.[17] Many other common drugs, including antidepressants, antihypertension drugs, and antianxiety drugs, have also been linked to cancer. Even over-the-counter supplements can be dangerous. According to an investigation by the New York State attorney, supplements from four national retailers—GNC, Target, Walgreens, and Walmart—were found *not* to contain the herb they were advertising but *were* subject to contamination and substitution with potential allergens not identified on the ingredient list.[18] I recommend only nutraceuticals, which are supplements that are high quality and sometimes only able to be prescribed by a practitioner. Quality is key. Find a few companies you trust and never buy over-the-counter supplements from big chain stores (see Recommended Resources in appendix D).

Carcinogens are also circulating in the air we breathe. There are 187 identified "hazardous air pollutants," some with obvious sources such as tobacco smoke, and others less obvious, such as volatile organic compounds (VOCs). VOCs, which have been linked to many cancers, enter our bodies through exposure to cleaning solutions, carpet, flooring, furniture, perfume, air fresheners, candles, craft supplies, and more. The VOC benzene is associated with leukemias and lymphomas and can be found in detergents, drugs, pesticides, sunscreens, and vehicle exhaust. It is frequently elevated near airports and gas stations.[19] According to the US-Citizens Aviation Watch Association, people living on the perimeter of Chicago's O'Hare airport have a 70 percent higher rate of cancer than the average Chicagoan.[20]

In addition to eating, drinking, and breathing carcinogens, we also absorb them through our skin. These carcinogens are mostly found in our clothing, cosmetics, and personal care products. When possible, buy organic clothing or used clothing that has been washed many times. When buying new

Carcinogens Commonly Found in Fabrics

- Azo dyes
- Dioxins
- Flame retardants
- Formaldehyde
- Heavy metals
- Pesticides
- Solvents

clothing, presoak and wash multiple times before wearing. Avoid anything that advertises itself as flame retardant, static resistant, stain resistant, or wrinkle free. These labels mean the material is full of carcinogens such as formaldehyde, Teflon, or nonylphenol ethoxylates and nonylphenols. The biggest offenders are flame-retardant pajamas, all the worse because children sleep in pajamas for eight to ten hours a night, sweating and absorbing these carcinogens into their skin. Buy fewer, better-quality clothes, and stick to natural fabrics like organic cotton, silk, wool, hemp, or linen.

Radiation is a carcinogen. Many studies have shown that radiation exposure increases the risk of cancer, including the risk of secondary cancers in children treated by radiation for their first malignancy. When your child has cancer, they may need to have imaging in the form of X-rays, CT scans, and MRIs that you can't easily avoid because these will be ways to monitor disease progression or regression. Discuss ways to decrease the radiation exposure with your child's oncology team, such as less frequent intervals or lower intensity (X-ray vs. CT scan). There are also ways to protect your child with nutrition and supplements before imaging (see chapter 3). Protecting your child as much as possible during treatment is key.

Electromagnetic frequencies (EMFs) given off by cell phones, computers, and cell towers is a newer, ubiquitous form of ambient exposure. Electronic devices such as iPads, cell phones, and laptops, are part of our children's

Consumer Products to Be Wary Of

- Body wash and soap
- Deodorant
- Hair products, including hair dye
- Lotion and body cream
- Makeup
- Nail polish
- Perfume
- Shampoo and conditioner
- Tampons and pads

The EWG runs a website called Skin Deep, which provides a list of personal care products with safety toxin ratings.

daily lives. The *Journal of Clinical Oncology* and *International Journal of Environmental Research and Public Health* found that, based on a meta-analysis of forty-six case-control studies, seventeen minutes on a cell phone per day over ten years is associated with a statistically significant, 60 percent increase in brain cancer.[21] If you purchase a phone for your child, teach them to keep it off their body, on airplane mode when possible, and turned off and away from the bedroom at night. You can completely turn your Wi-Fi router off at night or even hardwire your home. Invest in an EMF meter. Keep smart meters away from your child's bedroom. I have included a list of products that can help reduce the burden of EMF exposure in appendix D.

Finally—since we're on controversial topics—toxic burden can also come in the form of injections, such as IV "nutrition" and vaccines, which frequently include aluminum and formaldehyde. Be especially mindful when new vaccines come out on the market for which adverse reactions, especially in children with weakened immune systems, have not been adequately demonstrated.

The Microbiome

The human microbiota consists of up to 100 trillion symbiotic microbial cells, composed of bacteria, viruses, and fungi, and has more complexity than the human genome. The microbiome influences many aspects of human life, including the immune system, availability of nutrition, synthesis of vitamins, fat storage, and even behavior. A disrupted or unhealthy microbiome can contribute to cancer development, as well as influence the response to treatment.[22]

What leads to an unhealthy gut in a child? Our first exposure to "good" bacteria is through contact with our mom's vagina through a vaginal birth, which is why births by cesarean section are associated with the future development of numerous health conditions. In 2019, a study published in the scientific journal *Nature* analyzed almost 600 births and found that children born vaginally had very different gut microbes than those who were not.[23] A major study published in 2020 followed subjects for forty years and found that those born via cesarean section were significantly more likely to develop diabetes, celiac disease, arthritis, and inflammatory bowel disease—even several decades later.[24] Mayo Clinic researchers found that the administration of antibiotics to children younger than two is associated with multiple illnesses, including celiac disease, asthma, allergies, overweight and obesity,

ADHD, and atopic dermatitis.[25] Multiple studies are underway to investigate how our microbiome may have significant applications as a biomarker for diagnosis, prognosis, and management of certain cancers.

A disrupted microbiome can lead to many different illnesses. Those illnesses are then sometimes treated with drugs that further harm the microbiome and immune system, creating a vicious cycle that can contribute to a cancer diagnosis.[26] Altered gut microbiota is associated with resistance to chemotherapy drugs and immune checkpoint inhibitors; likewise, supplementing certain bacterial species can improve the response to anticancer drugs. You can also modulate the gut microbiota to enhance the effectiveness of your child's anticancer drugs. For example, key bacterial species (*Barnesiella intestinihominis* and *Enterococcus hirae*) have been identified that affect the chemotherapy drug cyclophosphamide. Removing these bacterial species results in drug resistance.[27]

Choose a pediatrician who does not overuse antibiotics. Fever reducers like acetaminophen (Tylenol) and ibuprofen (Advil) also disrupt the microbiome. (During my medical training, I was taught that any child with a fever must get acetaminophen every four hours and ibuprofen every six to eight hours. I had to unlearn this recommendation.) Also be wary of hand sanitizer. Most contain the carcinogen benzene and many also contain additional harmful (and sometimes unlisted) ingredients.[28] Bottom line: They are not needed. Teach your kids to wash their hands with water and nontoxic soap.

Additionally, you may discover that the use of probiotics during cancer treatment is a tricky subject with your child's oncologist. Probiotics can be phenomenal adjuncts in anticancer therapy, but in my experience, oncologists advise not to use them with chemotherapy because children are more susceptible to infection during treatment. Studies show, however, that probiotic bacteria can safely be administered in the setting of neutropenia (a lower-than-normal number of neutrophils). Even in the context of a hematopoietic stem cell transplant where a patient is neutropenic for a prolonged period of time, probiotics can be safely administered.[29] This is a risk-versus-benefit decision you should make with your integrative oncology practitioner.

My general rule is to use probiotics if the absolute neutrophil count is over 500. If it is under 500, I need to have a good reason, such as the ability of a particular strain of probiotics to mitigate chemotherapy resistance. Probiotics can also help with diarrhea, a common side effect of most anticancer therapies, and help restore the gut microbiome after treatment.[30] *Lacticaseibacillus rhamnosus* (formerly known as *Lactobacillus rhamnosus*) is an example of a bacteria that has been shown in multiple clinical studies to restore gut microbial balance. If you choose to go this route, it is a good idea to change up the probiotics every three months to introduce different types of beneficial bacteria to the body. (See chapter 11 for more on healing the gut post treatment.)

Immune Function

To understand how you can make your child's immune system better, let's first take a look at how the immune system works. The human immune system includes our lymph nodes, spleen, tonsils, thymus, and specialized cells, including natural killer cells (NK cells), B cells, T cells, and macrophages, which are part of the white blood cells made in the bone marrow. Although cancer cells appear similar to normal cells and can disguise themselves from immune system detection, a healthy immune system will be able to find and kill cancer cells. Cancer cells can paralyze the activity of the NK cells by producing an inflammatory cytokine reaction. Macrophages can eat cancer cells when they are working correctly.

You are reading this book, however, because your child's immune system was not operating well enough to stop the cancer cells. So, what could have caused your child's immune system impairment? There are many factors, but as I will discuss in chapter 6, nutrition plays a huge role. Our diet influences whether we have a healthy gut or a leaky gut. A leaky gut contributes to nutritional deficiencies. Medications also affect the health of our gut and therefore our immune system.

While there are times when prescription medications are necessary and even lifesaving, they can also cause immune system dysregulation. In addition to antibiotics, there are many other common offenders, including immunosuppressants, antacids, proton pump inhibitors, antipyretics (ibuprofen or acetaminophen), antianxiety and antidepressant medications, pain medications, constipation medications, and hormone replacement therapy. As you read through this list you may notice they are medications often used throughout most kids' cancer treatment or afterward, in survivorship. Let's take a quick look at the harm these medications cause to our immune system.

One of the most commonly used medications during cancer treatment is acetaminophen (Tylenol). Parents are told to use it when a child has a fever or pain. Most people know the damaging effects acetaminophen can have on the liver, but did you know that there is a regulatory effort in the state of California that is trying to classify it as a carcinogen?[31] In 2016, a professor of epidemiology at the University of Washington published a review of several studies that examined if using acetaminophen predisposes to cancer. He identified that there is a possible correlation with renal cell carcinoma, lymphoma, and leukemia.

Even if acetaminophen did not contribute to the development of your child's cancer, it certainly will not help during treatment. Acetaminophen is most often used for fevers, but fevers are the body's way of creating heat to help the immune system fight infection. Suppressing a fever means you are suppressing the body's ability to fight the illness. Acetaminophen also depletes glutathione, which is an antioxidant needed by your liver to detox. When a child is receiving chemotherapy, you want to do everything you can to support the liver detoxification pathways; acetaminophen does the opposite. In most cases it is safe for your child to have a fever during treatment. I will discuss safe therapies for your child's pain during treatment in chapter 9. When it is necessary to administer acetaminophen, you can also give your child liposomal glutathione or N-acetylcysteine to counter the glutathione-depleting effects of it.

It concerns me when I hear that a child doesn't get a fever in response to an infection. A fever is necessary for the immune system to battle infections. In Europe, cancer treatment often includes the stimulation of fever with therapies such as mistletoe (more on this in chapter 7).

Acid-reducing drugs, or proton pump inhibitors (PPIs), are another frequently prescribed medication during cancer treatment. This class of drugs is also not harmless and needs to be used with caution. Studies show an increased risk of kidney disease, osteoporosis, low magnesium and vitamin B12, pneumonia, and contracting *Clostridioides difficile* (*C. diff*) with the use of PPIs.[32] What's frustrating is that low magnesium and vitamin B12, infections, and *C. diff* are already concerns during cancer treatment. Incorrect use of PPIs can contribute to their occurrence. When my daughter, Zuza, had her bone marrow transplant, a PPI was ordered for daily use over the thirty-plus days of her hospital admission to help prevent pain from mucositis. In fact, studies show that the use of PPIs actually contributes to mucositis.[33] We chose not to use PPIs, and Zuza did not develop mucositis or pain.

Immunosuppressants can be lifesaving by preventing graft-versus-host disease or a life-threatening allergic reaction. Immunosuppressants are also used in some cancer treatments, such as treatment for ALL, and they are frequently used in anticancer therapy treatment. Common immunosuppressants include prednisone and dexamethasone; tacrolimus is a more intense variety. However, taking immunosuppressants presents significant risks; immunosuppressants . . . suppress your immune system. Risks include infection, malignancy, marrow suppression, cytopenia, cardiovascular disease, and diabetes. Short-term risks include high blood sugar, change in mood, nausea/vomiting, and insomnia. Prednisone is overused in conventional medicine. If your child has a rash or eczema, your pediatrician may prescribe steroid cream. I have met medical teams who preferred to have a patient on IV steroids as a preventative measure rather than risk any adverse effects of medications without the steroids. We will discuss alternatives to steroids and how to support the use of steroids in chapter 8.

Inflammation

Inflammation is a normal physiological process that promotes healing from an infection or injury. When you get a splinter, for example, your body's immune response creates inflammation in an attempt to rid your body of the foreign body (the splinter). It's important to understand that acute inflammation is protective. It is equally important to understand that inflammation becomes a problem when it is chronic. Chronic inflammation is a major precursor to cancer. The standard American diet contributes to chronic inflammation, and most processed foods are filled with highly inflammatory processed seed oils.

Dr. Nasha Winters states it best, in my opinion: "Inflammation is considered cancer's primary precursor. Genetic damage is the match that lights the fire, and inflammation the gas that sustains it."[34] Was there an inflammatory event that might have been a precursor to your child's diagnosis?

Chronic disease is the new epidemic, and the root of chronic disease is low-grade inflammation. Consider eczema, for example. You notice that your child has eczema, so you bring it up to your pediatrician and are sent home with a steroid cream. The steroid seems to work because the rash goes away while you are using it, but in fact, your child's skin is telling you that something is wrong. Treating the problem with an immunosuppressant only suppresses the immune system, exacerbating rather than healing the root of the problem. The root of the problem could be a leaky gut as a result of being a cesarean section baby or of using antibiotics, but instead of healing the gut and therefore the eczema, the steroid contributes to the problem because the immunosuppressant further damages your child's gut and immune system.

Inflammatory bowel disease provides another example of the mistreatment of an inflammatory process. Individuals diagnosed with ulcerative colitis or Crohn's disease have very specific precursors early in life. Intestinal bacteria are implicated in the cause of inflammatory bowel disease and because a cesarean section disrupts the normal bacteria colonization of the newborn's intestines, the risk of inflammatory bowel disease is significant for children between ages zero and fourteen who were born via cesarean section. In fact, the definition of *inflammatory bowel disease* is chronic inflammation of the digestive tract. This inflammation can be healed by healing the lining of the intestines; yet immunosuppressants are frequently used to suppress the immune system and contribute to further damage in the body.

In children, chronic inflammation can show up as a recurring rash or even persistent acne. Recurrent infections can also be related to chronic inflammation and should be addressed systemically, not just suppressed or treated with antibiotics.

Hormones

Hormonally driven cancers are on the rise among pediatric patients. I treated a fourteen-year-old girl with ovarian cancer, and many of my colleagues have reported similar instances. Until about the turn of the twentieth century, the average age of menarche (first period) was 16.5 years old. Today, the average age of menarche is 12.4. Later menarche is associated with a decreased risk of developing breast cancer.

Studies have shown that exposure to endocrine-disrupting chemicals is directly affecting hormonal development. In fact, newer research is showing that adolescents may exhibit higher sensitivity to even minimal concentrations of hormone-disrupting chemicals.[35] This is likely due to the closely related hormonal signals that are already active in the body as a natural part of puberty.

If your child consumes nonorganic animal products such as meat or dairy, they are being exposed to the sex hormones and steroids that are used on livestock. These added hormones accumulate in their bodies and can lead to hormonally driven cancers.

Both girls and boys, at increasingly younger ages, are being introduced to cosmetics and toiletries, which can contain endocrine-disrupting hormones unless explicitly verified as nontoxic. Consider a scenario involving a fourteen-year-old girl who follows a standard American diet; consumes nonorganic animal products; uses conventional makeup, deodorant, and perfume; and happens to possess an epigenetic SNP called COMT, which inhibits her ability to metabolize harmful estrogens effectively. Additionally, she is prescribed birth control by her pediatrician to manage acne and painful periods. This combination of factors is enough to increase the risk of developing ovarian or early breast cancer. The same concerns apply to boys who start using deodorant, cologne, and hair gel at a young age.

Stress and Emotional Health

Stress is very powerful and can significantly contribute to the development of cancer—even in kids. Prior to the COVID-19 pandemic, one in five youth suffered from depression or anxiety. The pandemic doubled that.[36] We are experiencing a global youth mental health crisis; suicide is the second leading cause of death among US children, followed by cancer.[37] Stress can increase your child's inflammation, spike their blood sugar, and suppress their immune system.

Kids have become part of our high-stress society, starting as early as kindergarten, or even before. Sports teams are competitive, schools pile on homework, and extracurricular activities leave kids no time to be kids. On top of that, social media makes many people, including children and teenagers, feel inadequate, and a highly competitive society projects parents' anxieties about their children's futures onto the children themselves.

The hypothalamic-pituitary-adrenal (HPA) axis is your body's stress response system. The HPA axis is a system of surveillance, protection, adaptation, and resilience, with the amygdala acting like a camera recording any sources of stress from either inside or outside the body. When the amygdala perceives stress, it sends a signal to the hypothalamus, which then sends a signal to the adrenals, which in turn release stress hormones like epinephrine and cortisol. This would be lifesaving if you were being chased by a vicious dog. But chronic stress caused by poor sleep, infections, poor diet, and negative thoughts can, over time, create a situation of a continual stress response through the HPA axis with little to no recovery. Constant release of cortisol can impact health through blood sugar dysregulation, weight gain, high blood pressure, and emotional instability.

Circadian rhythm disruption can also be a major stressor for children. Most children do not get enough sleep. Children ages four and under should be napping during the day and getting a full night's sleep of at least ten hours. From ages six to twelve, children should be getting at least nine hours of sleep. Teenagers need eight to ten hours. When your children are under four it is especially important to protect their sleep schedule and their naps.

Help your child maintain a before-bed routine that includes no electronics at least thirty minutes before bed; a dark, cool room; and no electronics in the room at night. Blue light exposure from a computer, TV, iPhone, or iPad can disrupt our circadian rhythm, causing a reduction in hormones and an increase in cortisol; we want the opposite before bed. Recent studies show that the blue light emitted by electronics not only stimulates the brain, inhibits melatonin secretion, and enhances adrenocortical hormone production but it also will destroy hormonal balance and directly affect our sleep quality. If your child must do homework on electronics before bed, have them wear blue-light-blocking glasses and program the device for automatic night mode.

A 2020 study concluded that chronic stress promotes cancer development through a variety of mechanisms.[38] In patients who already have cancer, studies have found that stress is linked to tumor growth.[39] Most families can look back at their child's life and identify a stressor that could have contributed to the cancer. Solutions often lie in lifestyle changes for the whole family. Having our kids involved in fewer activities is often positive, as long as they are not filling in those gaps with electronics. Sometimes the school a child attends is not the right fit and is a source of constant debilitating stress. While changing schools or homeschooling can be extraordinarily inconvenient or difficult, you must carefully weigh your child's well-being against all the other factors in your life. Breathwork and meditation can also be powerful tools for stress reduction.

CHAPTER 6

Develop a Nutrition Plan

OUR FOOD CRISIS IS REAL. IN THE UNITED STATES, THE MAJORITY OF grocery stores are filled with highly processed junk food, fast-food restaurants have lines at every hour of the day, and many people have little knowledge about what real food is let alone how to prepare it. The standard American diet not only lacks nutrients but also often contains known carcinogens.

Even parents who consider themselves to be feeding their families a "healthy" diet often have no idea what they are allowing into their children's bodies. For example, a child who eats a frozen waffle for breakfast is starting the day with bleached flour, processed seed oils, and high-fructose corn syrup. Lunch might be a salami and cheese sandwich on whole wheat bread, exposing them to the pesticides in the grain, processed seed oil in the bread, refined sugar, nitrates, antibiotics, and hormones. Spaghetti and meatballs with spinach salad for dinner is more of the same, unless the spinach is organic and the meat is from grass-fed animals raised by a conscientious farmer.

Where is the healthy fat needed for brain health? Where is the variety of plants and quality proteins for cell growth and healthy function?

For a child with cancer, nutrition is the foundation of healing, so starting today, it is time to get serious about your family's nutrition and the quality of food coming into your home. By the end of this chapter, you'll have an understanding of how to start your child on a nutrient-dense diet with the macronutrient profile that is the least conducive to cancer growth and also protective to healthy cells.

But first things first: If you do nothing else, feed your family real food. Real food is easy to recognize: It has one ingredient. From there, the next step is to feed your family organic food, free of pesticides and herbicides. This is more complicated due to a confusing USDA certification system. While your best bet will generally be certified organic food as opposed to food without a certified organic label, that's not universally true. Not all certified organic food is healthy; a lot of packaged organic food is full of refined sugar and other ingredients that you don't want in your child's body whether those ingredients are organic or not. Those organic cookies? Leave them on the supermarket shelf.

On the other hand, a lot of excellent healing foods won't be labeled organic because, just like that carrot out of your home garden won't be labeled organic, some farmers who use organic methods choose not to obtain the costly organic certification. So just because something isn't *labeled* organic doesn't mean it *isn't* organic, especially if you're buying from a small, local producer. The bottom line? Always buy real food as locally as possible, get to know your farmers, ask questions, and when in doubt, spend the extra money to buy certified organic products free of herbicides and pesticides.

Every year the Environmental Working Group (EWG) releases its "Dirty Dozen" list. These are the twelve fruits and vegetables with the highest amount of pesticide residue. Pay attention to these yearly lists and always (at minimum) look for organic options for everything on the Dirty Dozen list. You can sign up for annual updates at the EWG website.[1] Each year, the list is

The EWG's Dirty Dozen (2023)

1. Strawberries
2. Spinach
3. Kale, collards, and mustard greens
4. Peaches
5. Pears
6. Nectarines
7. Apples
8. Grapes
9. Bell and hot peppers
10. Cherries
11. Blueberries
12. Green beans

How to Wash Produce

Fill a container with water to cover the produce. If possible, use filtered water and do not use a plastic container. Add one teaspoon of baking soda for each two cups of water or one table-spoon of apple cider vinegar for each two cups of water. Allow the produce to soak for twelve to fifteen minutes. Then scrub.[2]

similar. (Strawberries and apples are almost always on the Dirty Dozen list.) Avoid pick-your-own operations unless they are organic. The Dirty Dozen are great foods to grow in your own home garden.

The EWG also publishes a "Clean Fifteen." These are the fruits and vegetables with the least amount of pesticide residue, so if you must buy some foods conventionally, the Clean Fifteen would be a better option than the Dirty Dozen. Don't fool yourself though: There will still likely be pesticides and herbicides present. In fact, even organic fruits and vegetables often have some level of pesticides present. For this reason, please wash all your produce, whether organic or not.

In addition to making better choices around fruits and vegetables, it's important to pay attention to grains and beans. A 2014 study found that up to 63 percent of bread products contain pesticide residue.[3] The EWG has found pesticides in more than 95 percent of oat products, including children's cereal.[4] Chickpeas, which you might feed your child as part of a healthy hummus snack, are often heavily sprayed with the herbicide glyphosate (see below).[5] Sadly, even an organic wheat farm might be situated between conventional farms, subjecting it to pesticide drift.

Is the extra cost to buy organic worth it? Multiple studies suggest that it is. For instance, a 2006 study published in *Environmental Health Perspectives* showed that feeding children an organic diet for only five days provided reduced exposure to the organophosphorus pesticides commonly used in agriculture.[6] A 2021 study published in *Neuroscience News* demonstrated that an organic diet is linked to higher intelligence and better cognitive development in children.[7]

A Word about Glyphosate

In my opinion, the most devastating chemical to enter our world was glyphosate, sold under the trade name Roundup. In 1974, Roundup was brought to the market for residential use. By 2017, a decades-long cover-up of glyphosate's toxicity was unearthed, and in 2018 a groundbreaking lawsuit filed by a groundskeeper named Dewayne "Lee" Johnson, who claimed that acute glyphosate exposure resulted in his non-Hodgkin lymphoma, resulted in $78 million in damages paid by Roundup's manufacturer, Monsanto.

In the United States, Monsanto (now owned by Bayer) stopped selling Roundup for residential use in 2023, but commercial use continues unabated. That means Roundup will continue to be applied in parks, schoolyards, even nature centers, and it will continue to be in our food, including as a desiccant at harvest time (meaning the rain won't be washing it off after application). Although Roundup has been banned in more than twenty countries, our nation's food supply continues to be doused in it.

In my medical practice, I test my patients for glyphosate toxicity, as well as other herbicides and pesticides. I have never had a patient with zero glyphosate exposure. In fact, there is no such thing as zero percent glyphosate exposure anymore, even among those of us who exclusively eat organic foods. Glyphosate sneaks into our lives and our bodies every day. But we can dramatically reduce our exposure by buying organic.

Another benefit of buying organic is that you will be avoiding genetically modified foods. Genetic modification is extremely common in staple crops such as corn, soybeans, potatoes, canola, apples, alfalfa, and much more. Not all non-GMO food is organic, but all organic food is non-GMO. When in doubt, look for a non-GMO sticker or label.

Dietary Guidelines

It would be wonderful if feeding your ailing child a healing diet were as simple as buying organic food and washing it well. I'm sorry to say that it's not. Here is where I begin to deviate, in a big way, from conventional wisdom you may have heard. I do not believe that the United States Department of Agriculture (USDA) Dietary Guidelines will lead your child (or anyone else, for that matter) to health and healing.[8] These guidelines, in my opinion and the opinion of many experts, are not based on sound nutrition. The so-called food pyramid recommends a diet high in grains and carbohydrates, with fat-free or low-fat dairy, fortified soybean beverages as alternatives to dairy, lean meats, vegetable oils rather than animal fats, and refined sugar in moderation.

By comparison, I prescribe a more "traditional" diet, such as the diet recommended by the Weston A. Price Foundation as well as other traditional food experts and organizations. The foundations of this type of diet are animal foods, including muscle meat, organs, bones, fat, and skin. It is essential that the animals be ethically raised—*not* confined to a feedlot and fed grains supplemented with hormones and antibiotics—by a knowledgeable farmer practicing sound regenerative grazing practices. This type of diet also includes raw, full-fat dairy; properly prepared grains, nuts, legumes, and seeds (by which I mean sprouted, soaked, and/or sour-leavened); as well as organic, local, seasonal fruits and vegetables, prepared properly or fermented; and *small* amounts of natural sweeteners such as raw honey.

This type of diet is not a fad! (If anything, the USDA guidelines are a fad.) For tens of thousands of years humans have subsisted on traditional diets. With the arrival of mass production of industrial foods, the human diet changed dramatically and rapidly, and in recent decades we have seen a massive uptick in lifestyle-related diseases, including in our children. This is a tragedy. Our children don't have time to wait for regulatory bodies to promote and police industrial agriculture. As parents, we need to do this ourselves—starting now.

In this book, I refer to Foundation Nutrition, which are simple guidelines, very similar to what you might find from the Weston A. Price Foundation or in a ketogenic diet, that form the foundation of a nutrient-dense healing diet. If you are familiar with the Weston A. Price diet, you'll know that soaked and sprouted grains and legumes make up a significant part of that way of eating. A fundamental difference between the Weston A. Price diet and my Foundation Nutrition guidelines, is that I recommend limiting legumes, and removing all grains as much as possible. The reasons for this are multiple. For the most part, grains and legumes are some of the foods on the market most contaminated by glyphosate. They are also very high in carbohydrates. While soaking and sprouting grains and legumes makes them more digestible, it does not reduce the carbohydrate content or the glyphosate levels. High-carbohydrate foods should be limited in the foundational diet of a child with pediatric cancer. In general, a grain-free and legume-free diet also tends to be denser in nutrients per calorie.

If you are able to carefully source glyphosate-free gluten-free grains and legumes, and you are able to prepare them properly by soaking and fermenting them, these food items can be occasionally included in the Foundation Nutrition diet. They are not a "never" food in the way that high-fructose corn syrup is, but they are rather something I would use occasionally if I enjoyed the food item enough that the trouble of sourcing and preparation was worth it for me. For example, a small occasional slice of homemade organic sourdough bread made from a low-gluten, ancient grain like Red Fife is not in the same category as a store-bought slice of wheat bread. However, your child will get all the nutrients they need from Foundation Nutrition without going through the trouble of making fresh sourdough bread from fresh-milled ancient grains—so I see this as more of an optional additive rather than a part of your foundational diet.

When a child receives a diagnosis of cancer or a recurrence, I recommend tweaking the Foundation Nutrition that everyone should be eating by eliminating natural sugars and increasing the amounts of healthy fats. I refer to this tweak as Level 1 Nutrition. There may also be times when you want to further restrict your child's diet. Level 2 Nutrition is essentially a ketogenic diet, intended to put your child into ketosis. Level 2 Nutrition isn't an easy diet to follow, especially for children and for families under the profound stress that a cancer diagnosis can bring, so I recommend putting your child into ketosis only under certain circumstances, such as prior to an inpatient stay when they will need as much nutritional healing as possible to help them undergo the rigors of chemotherapy, bone marrow transplants, or other treatments that carry serious and intense risks and side effects.

Before I go any further, there's an important subject I need to address: There is a large movement focused on beating cancer with a vegan diet. It is true that processed, antibiotic- and chemical-filled meats should be avoided by everyone; it is also true that this kind of meat can contribute to cancer. I am *not* promoting processed, antibiotic- and chemical-filled meats. However, for pediatric cancer, animal protein is necessary. In fact, any child going through conventional cancer treatment needs *lots* of protein because protein is easily lost during treatment. Pediatric cancer patients need complete proteins for the best functioning of their immune system and to help prevent and or treat cachexia (muscle wasting and extreme weight loss). Pasture-raised, grass-finished organic beef, eggs, poultry, wild game, and wild fish have the necessary proteins to support a developing child and especially a developing child going through harsh conventional cancer treatment. A vegan diet for young children includes major health risks because it has an inadequate supply of quality protein as well as not enough of the following: long-chain fatty acids, iron, zinc, vitamin D3, iodine, calcium, and vitamin B12 (all of which can be found in quality animal protein). Therefore, well-sourced, organic animal protein should be part of a child's nutrition during cancer treatment and after, as their body heals from cancer treatment.

Foundation Nutrition

The following are simple guidelines that form the foundation of a nutrient-dense healthy diet for your family and your child.

Animal foods, especially organ meats. Organ meats are the most nutrient-dense part of the animal. If a child is squeamish about eating organ meats, these can often be mixed into dishes such as meatballs or stews. If your child has a nasogastric or gastric tube, organ meats can be blended and incorporated into their diet this way. Source grass-fed and -finished meats from a local grocer or market, or better yet, identify a local farmer who raises animals on pasture and can sell meat directly.

Stocks and broths. Meat stocks and bone broths from well-sourced animals can be incredibly healing. I recommend incorporating stocks and broths into your child's diet as much as possible. They are full of minerals, collagen, and glycine to support and heal the gut. Homemade stocks and broths from well-sourced animals is best.

High-quality fats. Healthy fats include butter, ghee, tallow, duck fat, lard, coconut oil, extra virgin olive oil, and avocado oil. The best fats are animal fats from local farmers. Supplement this with organic quality fats in glass bottles from a local grocer.

Organic full-fat dairy. For kids who can tolerate cow's milk, raw milk is best (although it can be tricky to source). For kids who do not tolerate dairy, I recommend goat or sheep's milk, including yogurt and cheese (as well as homemade nut milks). If you can't get raw, full-fat dairy from a local farmer, the next best option is organic full-fat dairy from a local grocer.

Organic, local, and seasonal produce. This will depend on where you live. I live in the Midwest, so in the spring we eat a lot of mushrooms, chives, lettuce, and other greens. In summer, our diet includes more tomatoes, strawberries, asparagus, and peaches. In autumn, we eat a lot of melons, apples, pears, and sweet potatoes. And in the winter, we enjoy pumpkin, parsnips, and tropical fruit in season. See appendix D for resources for other regions. Local, organic produce from a farmers' market is excellent, and the best produce will come from your own garden (assuming you do not treat it with any chemicals, or live next to someone who does).

Salt. Include mineral-rich unrefined salt mined from the sea in your child's diet. I recommend Himalayan pink salt, and REAL salt.

Natural sweeteners (optional). In small amounts, local honey, maple syrup, coconut sugar, dates and date sugar, blackstrap molasses, monk fruit, and organic stevia can be incorporated into recipes.

Soaked, sprouted, organic grains, legumes, nuts, and seeds (optional). This includes genuine sourdough bread, soaked and washed rice, soaked glyphosate-free oatmeal, soaked and sprouted organic gluten-free grains, and grain-free alternatives like organic almond flour, cassava flour, and coconut flour. If you choose to include these items, it is better to choose organic. The best, but still optional, way to consume these items is to source them as organic and sprouted. If you choose to consume grain flours they should be sourced from farms that are not within a couple of miles of nonorganic farms.

Hydration is a very important part of healing and detoxification. During treatment, your child's kidneys will be coping with many toxins, and the key to supporting the kidneys so the toxins pass out of the body is hydration. Roughly speaking, I recommend your child drink half their body weight (in pounds) in fluid ounces each day. For example, if your child weighs fifty pounds, they should drink approximately twenty-five ounces of water per day. (During inpatient visits, hydration is usually one of the IVs your child will be hooked up to. It's important to ask for normal saline rather than sugar water/dextrose.)

That said, not all water is equal. Unfortunately, both municipal and well water often hide toxins, including glyphosate. I recommend testing your water and investing in a high-quality filter for your home. You can purchase either a whole-house filter or an under-the-sink reverse osmosis filter and separate filters for the bath and shower. Avoid drinking water from plastic bottles. Is there a better water than filtered water? Possibly. Although more research needs to be done, studies have shown that deuterium-depleted water can inhibit cancer growth.[9]

Not Foundation Nutrition

The following are foods to avoid when maintaining a nutrient-dense healthy diet.

Vegetable oils. Canola oil, corn oil, soybean oil, grape-seed oil, peanut oil, safflower oil, sunflower oil, margarine and other butter alternatives, vegetable oil, and vegetable shortening and other highly processed (and usually inexpensive) oils. (Note that grape-seed oil is different than grape-seed extract.)

Refined sweeteners. High-fructose corn syrup, granulated sugar, brown sugar, powdered sugar, juice concentrates, and artificial sweeteners such as aspartame, sucralose, and saccharin.

Genetically modified corn products and soy additives. High-fructose corn syrup, corn oil, cornmeal, cornstarch, soy lecithin, and soybean oil.

Processed, packaged foods. Premade meals, packaged chips or pretzels, frozen snacks, protein bars, conventional breads, cookies, cakes, and more.

Vegan fake foods. Plant-based milks and vegan cheeses, meats, eggs, and anything made chemically to taste like the real thing.

Industrial, ultra-pasteurized low-fat dairy. Pasteurization destroys the important enzymes necessary to support our bodies in being able to digest milk or other dairy products. In addition, there are often harmful additives and vegetable oils in many industrial, low-fat dairy products. We *want* the fat in the milk, as this is where the vitamins are and calcium is naturally.

Level 1 Nutrition

Now that we have established the difference between a standard American diet and Foundation Nutrition for your family, let's talk about how and why to tweak it. There can be a number of reasons why you might want to tweak your child's Foundation Nutrition by eliminating certain foods and increasing the quantities of other foods. It could be that your child has been diagnosed with cancer but you haven't yet found an integrative oncology practitioner, and you want to boost their nutrition as you await further guidance. Or your child has a secondary illness, such as a cold or stomach bug, or is simply feeling unwell. Or your child has completed conventional treatment and it's time to detox and start healing the gut.

Tweaking Foundation Nutrition to Level 1 Nutrition is relatively simple: Adjust macros by focusing on more fats and proteins and reducing carbohydrates. As you transition to Level 1 Nutrition, you will remove all grain, including anything made from grain flours (breads, crackers, pasta) and rice. Replace this with nongrain organic carbohydrates in *small* quantities, such as soaked and sprouted organic millet, buckwheat, quinoa, and amaranth. You can also use cassava, coconut, and almond flour. In addition to removing grains, also remove beans (even organic and properly soaked and prepared beans).

At the same time, increase healthy fats, including avocado, MCT (medium chain triglyceride) oil, organic butter, and ghee, and also increase protein intake. Focus on well-sourced and grass-finished animal meats and quality protein powders. Increase organic vegetables, especially cruciferous vegetables such as broccoli and cauliflower. Increase probiotic-rich foods such as sauerkraut, kefir, and kimchi. Focus on organic and seasonal fruit as a condiment to your meals rather than serving these in very large amounts.

Level 2 Nutrition (Ketosis)

Cancer thrives on glucose, so to starve cancer cells, you need to restrict sugar and carbohydrates.[10] When you do this, the body flips a metabolic switch, enabling it to use stored fat as fuel instead of glucose. Ketone bodies are produced in the liver and distributed all over the body for energy. Ketosis therefore typically begins with either a short fast or significant reduction in carbohydrates. While starvation is not an option, we can mimic the benefits of a short-term starvation state through fasting or a fasting mimicking diet. This starvation mimicry can stress tumor tissue and help eliminate dysfunctional cells.[11]

My experience suggests that kids can have an easier time during treatment when they follow a metabolic therapy called ketosis. *Ketosis* is a process that happens when your body does not have enough carbohydrates to burn for energy, so it burns fat and makes ketones, which are used for fuel instead. Ketosis is a metabolic state. It is not a fad diet. There are different types of ketogenic diets. A ketogenic diet is any diet that can help you achieve ketosis.

There are many potential benefits to ketosis during treatment, including protecting healthy cells from radiation or chemotherapy damage, slowing tumor growth, antitumor effects, prolonging survival time, decreasing side effects of radiation and chemotherapy, reducing drug toxicity (from chemotherapy/radiation), and offering a better quality of life.[12] Multiple animal and human studies have demonstrated how effective ketosis can be during treatment for multiple pediatric cancers, including brain tumors, neuroblastoma, and certain solid tumors.

If you are considering putting your child into ketosis by moving from Level 1 Nutrition to Level 2 Nutrition, I urge you to work with a qualified practitioner. A typical ketogenic diet includes a moderate amount of protein and about 70 percent of total calories from fat. This is enough to get into nutritional ketosis with blood ketone levels above 0.5 millimoles per liter. However, for a therapeutic ketosis during chemotherapy and radiation, we want more ketone bodies and blood ketone levels between 2.5 and 6 millimoles per liter. Before you get overwhelmed, be aware that therapeutic ketosis is generally easier for kids to achieve than adults.

It is important to understand the distinction between the "keto diet" you may hear about in magazines and the internet, which includes things like diet soda, sugar-free Jell-O, and all kinds of mass-produced "keto snacks" and the *metabolic state of ketosis*—which is what we are trying to achieve here, in Level 2 Nutrition, while following a nutrient-dense and toxin-free diet.

Moving forward, when I refer to a ketogenic diet, please understand that I am not referring to the trendy "keto diet" I just described; I am referring to the metabolic therapy of consuming a diet low in carbohydrates and higher in fat, with the goal of putting the body into the metabolic state of ketosis. The foods consumed while on a ketogenic diet should be the nutrient-dense foods described here, not simply "low-carb foods."

How do you transition your child to ketosis? First work on Foundation Nutrition. When you're ready, transition to Level 1 Nutrition by removing grains and legumes. When you're ready again, transition to Level 2 Nutrition by removing fruit and other high-carbohydrate foods, such as millet, buckwheat, and quinoa, while increasing healthy fat intake. Level 2 Nutrition will put your child into the metabolic state of ketosis.

Within the scope of ketogenic diets, 3:1 and 4:1 ketogenic diets are very strict. A 4:1 ketogenic diet contains four grams of fat for every one gram of protein and carbohydrates combined. A 3:1 ketogenic diet contains three grams of fat for every one gram of protein and carbohydrates combined.

Sometimes, your practitioner may recommend you transition further into ketosis by following a 3:1 or 4:1 ketogenic diet.

If you are breastfeeding, just continue. Exclusively breastfed infants are in a state of mild ketosis anyway because breast milk is high in fat. If your infant is on formula, I recommend making your own ketogenic formula or using a commercial ketogenic formula. If you want your infant to be in a higher state of ketosis, you can continue to breastfeed while incorporating a ketogenic formula to raise the ketone levels.[13]

It is a good idea to monitor daily net carbohydrates, which are total grams of carbohydrate minus grams of fiber. Many kids can attain ketosis by keeping daily net carbohydrates below fifty grams. The Cronometer app can help you track macronutrients. Use its keto calculator, starting with either relaxed or moderate. It will give you a recommendation for amounts of healthy fats, protein, and net carbohydrates to achieve ketosis.

There are a few ways to test if your child is in the metabolic state of ketosis. Blood ketone meters are the most accurate, but you can also use urine sticks or breath tests. I prefer blood glucose and ketone meters and recommend the Keto-Mojo meter.

When transitioning into ketosis, it is important to keep a few things in mind. First, hydration is key. Add electrolytes daily. Supplement magnesium if your child becomes constipated. Keep an eye on glucose and ketone levels. If your child is undergoing inpatient treatment, make sure they are receiving a normal saline IV without any dextrose, and be aware that liquid medications often contain sugar and artificial colors. Steroids such as prednisone will increase your child's blood sugar and have the potential to take them out of ketosis, so consider using exogenous ketones if steroids are required. I recommend liquid ketones from a company called Ketone IQ. We dose ¼ to a full 2 ounce bottle depending on the child's weight and existing ketone level. Test their ketones thirty to sixty minutes later and decide if you need additional dosing.

Your child should not follow a ketogenic diet without the support of a ketogenic trained practitioner if they have liver disease or elevated liver enzymes, a history of surgery affecting the gastrointestinal tract, type 1 diabetes, type 2 diabetes on medications, gallbladder disease, kidney disease, and cachexia. For these reasons and others, it is extremely important that you work with an experienced metabolic practitioner and communicate with your child's oncology team.

Many side effects of ketosis are transitional, the most common of which is constipation. You can alleviate constipation by keeping your child hydrated with water and salted bone broth; increase ketosis-friendly foods that have a laxative effect, such as MCT oil; add probiotics if your child is not neutropenic; consider magnesium citrate before bed; keep your child walking; and consider abdominal massage or abdominal cupping.

Many children will also experience a set of side effects known as the "keto flu." Symptoms can include headache, body aches, constipation, and irritability. This is the body adapting to the metabolic shift; hydration with water and electrolytes will help reduce symptoms. Supplementing with 20 milligrams per kilogram L-carnitine two to three times per day with food and 500 milligrams vitamin B5 once a day with food can also be beneficial.

As the body shifts from using sugar as fuel to using fat as fuel, your child may also experience hypoglycemia, or low blood sugar. If they seem irritated, weak, confused, or shaky, check their glucose and their blood pressure. If glucose is below 60 milligrams per deciliter, give them a few sips of orange juice or apple juice and recheck it in thirty minutes. Hypoglycemia will resolve after a few weeks after the body adjusts. They may also experience some muscle cramping, which can be the result of dehydration or electrolyte imbalance. Again, hydration with water and electrolytes or salted bone broth should help.

If your child has elevated liver enzymes or any liver issues whatsoever, it is imperative that you work with an experienced practitioner to transition them into ketosis. The ketogenic diet can be healing to the liver (as it is for fatty liver disease), but you must also monitor your child's lab results and general health more closely.

Likewise, if your child has any gallbladder issues, it is imperative to work with an experienced practitioner and proceed with caution. Gallbladder issues are less common in children than in adults, but a well-functioning gallbladder (or key supplements, such as digestive enzymes) is needed for the body to handle the increased amount of fat in a ketogenic diet.

Some parents wonder if their child should be in ketosis throughout the entire treatment. This is something to discuss with your integrative practitioner, but in general, the answer is that it depends. If your child has a brain tumor, there is quite a lot of evidence demonstrating the value of ketosis, and you might consider keeping your child in ketosis.[14] If your child has ALL, however, is in remission, is only on oral chemo, and is doing well, then you might move back to Level 1 Nutrition. The most important time for a child to be in ketosis is during IV chemo infusions and days of radiation therapy. For example, if a child has three days of IV chemo infusions every three weeks, then you might transition your child into ketosis the day before the IV infusion, the day of, and next day, and then allow them to come out of ketosis until the next cycle. There are many ways of using this therapy.

Fasting is another tool that can be helpful. Research shows that it can reduce side effects of chemotherapy, enhance quality of life, protect healthy cells, and slow down tumor progression.[15] Patients will often fast for three days around their infusion, from day −1 (the day prior to infusion) to day 2 after infusion. I recommend fasting only for older kids who are capable of being a part of this decision for themselves. For young children, fasting can be hard both on them and on you as their caregiver. In addition, if you try to have your young child fast, your medical team will likely push back. I don't recommend getting into an argument with your medical team over fasting, as younger kids can mimic fasting through entering into ketosis.

When fasting, I recommend drinking plenty of fluids (half your child's body weight in ounces per day), mostly in the form of vegetable broth, water, and tea, with an emphasis on hydration and electrolyte support. Coconut oil or other plant oils can be given to support ketogenic metabolism without compromising the fasting state. Fasting is best done on a three-week cycle, with more caution and modifications needed for patients on a two-week cycle.

The best way to do fasting around chemotherapy is to fast after breakfast the day before, fast the day of, and fast till dinner the day after. However, this is assuming that the chemotherapy is only one day per week, and this is usually not the case. Therefore instead of fasting for children, I usually recommend a fasting mimicking diet (which is a ketogenic diet) so that they can eat through chemotherapy or radiation but still get the benefit of fasting. Between fasts, emphasize nutritionally dense, high-protein foods to aid in recovery between cycles.

In the same way it is possible to enter ketosis on a keto fad diet of diet soda and low-carbohydrate processed food, you can also attain a state of ketosis through a carnivore, vegan, or vegetarian diet. It is very attainable, but you won't necessarily be getting the nutrients the body needs. Again, it is essential to work with an experienced practitioner who can guide you along the way.

There are also some challenges you might face in putting your child on an "extreme" diet. This can include skepticism from the oncology team or your family and friends; concern about too much weight loss (cachexia); pushback from the hospital nutritionist; changing a family's and a child's eating habits, often dramatically; and more.

Skepticism from the Oncology Team

It takes new therapies an average of seventeen years to move from research to practice. That means researchers might have found a safe and effective treatment, but patients will have to wait an average of seventeen years before they have access to it. Your child doesn't have seventeen years. And if the therapy doesn't promise lucrative profits, it might languish in obscurity forever.

The ketogenic diet has been used and studied for decades in pediatric epilepsy patients, including in infants as young as six weeks old.[16] Ketogenic diets have also been studied in pediatric cancer patients (as well as adult cancer patients) and have been demonstrated safe and beneficial.[17] You have the right to choose your child's nutrition. You do not need anyone's permission to cut sugar and grains from your child's diet during treatment. Every time my daughter underwent treatment, I notified her medical team that she would be on a ketogenic diet and that I needed her IV nutrition and anything the chemotherapy was mixed with (this is common) to be free of sugar. Her doctors would check for hypoglycemia for a few days and then, seeing that it wasn't an issue, stopped checking.

Many studies, including systematic reviews and meta-analyses, support the use of ketogenic metabolic therapy for cancer.[18] In addition to an antitumor benefit, ketosis during IV chemotherapy or radiation treatment helps protect healthy cells, reduce toxicity, and reduce side effects.

Weight Loss (Cachexia)

Many parents who have children with cancer fear that their child will lose too much weight while battling the disease. This is known as cachexia, a multifactorial disease characterized by weight loss and an imbalance in metabolic regulation. Many factors can contribute to cachexia, including altered protein and energy metabolism, loss of appetite, and chronic inflammation. Cachexia accounts for up to 20 percent of cancer-related deaths.

While cachexia is a legitimate concern, the best prevention is not a diet of sugar and grain. In fact, feeding your child sugar and grain and processed foods during treatment can *contribute* to cachexia. How do you know if your child is starting to get into the danger zone? When weight loss is combined with a drop below normal in protein and albumin labs, cachexia may be at play. How do we reverse it? We remove sugar and grain and add in lots of healthy fats. Sound familiar? Yes, we put the child on a ketogenic diet. Appendix B includes recipes for anti-cachexia formula and smoothies. You can also give your child a teaspoon of MCT oil every few hours to help counteract malnutrition and the early signs of cachexia. Of course, you should always work with a professional to address cachexia.

Pushback from the Hospital Nutritionist

Pediatric cancer patients need excellent nutrition, so it's unfortunate that the nutritionists on pediatric cancer inpatient units typically give very poor nutritional advice. When I met my daughter's inpatient nutritionist, she was drinking a Diet Coke. She explained to me that calories are calories, and recommended feeding my daughter PediaSure—a product whose ingredients are as follows: water, corn maltodextrin, blend of vegetable oils (soy, high oleic safflower), sugar, milk protein concentrate, cocoa powder (processed with alkali), soy protein isolate.

Other than the water, none of these ingredients is healthy for any child, let alone a child going through cancer. If your child's nutritionist recommends foods containing ingredients like these, that alone should make you question any further recommendations. Standard-of-care nutritionists and dieticians attend schools that promote the USDA food guidelines; therefore, it is unreasonable to expect an inpatient nutritionist to work outside this paradigm. We already know these are poor guidelines.

To be fair, however, I have worked with some excellent inpatient nutritionists. In my experience, it is best to be honest about your nutrition plan and involve your oncology team, your integrative practitioner, and your nutritionist. Some hospitals even have a nutritionist skilled in the ketogenic diet, usually because they have been working with pediatric epilepsy patients. You can ask for, or even hire, a consulting nutritionist for additional support.

The Bottom Line

When a child is seriously ill, it's not uncommon for one parent to explore every possible therapy, while the other parent resists anything outside of conventional oncological recommendations. Even if you and your spouse are both on board, you may encounter disapproval from other members of your family. While you and your spouse need to get on the same page, remember that the responsibility is yours together, and therefore the decisions are yours together. It is not your nutritionist's or your clinician's place to convince you that you must follow their recommendation if you do not feel comfortable or convinced by what they've said. Professionals may be extremely dedicated, but remember that it's your child, and you are the one who must reckon with whatever decisions you make on your child's behalf.

Feeding Tubes

Some children will need a feeding tube during treatment. In other cases, it may not be strictly necessary but your child may benefit. If your child has difficulty eating or drinking, or suffers from bloating, nausea, or vomiting, a feeding tube can diminish discomfort and improve their quality of life and make it much easier to supply your child with nutrient-dense, healing foods. Your child's oncology team will likely make recommendations one way or another, but the decision is yours as a parent to make. Of course, if they are old enough, your child's feelings should be taken into consideration as well.

The least invasive option is a nasogastric (NG) tube, which is inserted through the nose, down the esophagus, and into the stomach. It takes about a minute to insert and must be replaced once a month. Occasionally, children will throw it up, and it will need to be replaced.

Another option for children who will be in intensive treatment for a long time, such as for a bone marrow transplant, is a gastric tube (G tube), which requires surgery and therefore a period of recovery as well. Some patients who start chemotherapy right after diagnosis may be too neutropenic and at risk of infection for a G tube.

I know it can be extraordinarily difficult for parents to see their child with a feeding tube, but my opinion is that the benefits frequently outweigh the drawbacks, including the risk of malnutrition. With a feeding tube, you eliminate the stress of low appetite, your child not wanting to eat certain foods, and having to take supplements. I recommend a G tube called the Mic-Key Button.

Keep the G tube clean with soap and water. If your child's skin begins to get irritated, you can apply barrier cream and gauze and/or diluted tea tree oil, or give your child Epsom salt baths with a few drops of tea tree oil. Alternatively, you can make a hypertonic saline dressing by mixing two teaspoons of table salt with one cup of warm water. Soak clean gauze in the solution, squeeze out the excess, and then place the gauze around the feeding tube for five to ten minutes up to five times a day. Always communicate with your child's G tube team for any troubleshooting if there are issues.

I encourage parents to place a feeding tube before treatment begins. An NG tube is less invasive and easier to insert, while a G tube is easier to use on a long-term basis. Another advantage of a feeding tube is that you can make your own formula, thinning it as necessary with nourishing bone broth or herbal tea (or water). When my daughter was undergoing treatment, I made "Super Soup" formula once a week, freezing it in breast milk bags, and then thawing and using it for the rest of the week. (You can find my Super Soup recipe in appendix B.)

Transitioning Your Child Out of Ketosis

If you've managed to get your child into ketosis, how long is it ideally beneficial for them to stay there? It depends. It might make sense to keep a child with a brain tumor on a ketogenic diet—or at least a very low-carbohydrate, high-quality high-fat diet—for several years, whereas it might make sense to keep a child with acute myeloid leukemia in ketosis only for several months of active treatment. The benefits of ketosis must be weighed against the family's capacity to sustain such a diet, as well as the child's own agency and desires. As you will likely feel over and over, making these kinds of difficult decisions requires a combination of parental intuition, the advice of your metabolic clinician, and an accounting of the benefits versus costs.

For children whose labs and trifecta numbers are good (see chapter 3 and appendix A "Trifecta Labs") and who are ready to move on from conventional oncology treatment, I recommend transitioning back to Level 1 Nutrition by reintroducing some nutrient-dense carbohydrates such as organic millet and sweet potato, along with seasonal fruits, while still restricting grains and gluten to allow for gut healing and detoxification. While many pediatric cancer patients will then be well served to transition all the way back to Foundation Nutrition, some may need longer with Level 1 Nutrition. In my experience, gut healing can take years. Puberty is another important time when you might want to consider Level 1 Nutrition. During this time, children need more protein and healthy fats to support their hormonal changes and this can be a vulnerable time for relapse. Up to 90 percent of childhood cancer survivors have late effects. With good nutrition, I believe we can reduce the risk.

———

I hope it's clear that good nutrition is essential to thriving with cancer. The standard American diet *contributes* to disease, including cancer. By the time you get your hands on this book, your child may already be in the midst of treatment. It's never too late to learn about real nutrition! Dietary changes should involve the entire family, not only to support your child battling cancer, but as an investment in the long-term health and well-being of everyone in the family. The value of healing foods after conventional treatment can make a tremendous difference if your child relapses or experiences late effects. Your child will be stronger and have more capacity to withstand additional treatment further down the road, if necessary.

Do my dietary recommendations guarantee remission for your child? No. I dearly wish I could promise that, but I can't. What I can say is that I've worked with many patients and their families, and lived through this with my own daughter, and I know firsthand that Foundation Nutrition results in less suffering, more joy, and fewer side effects. Your child's oncology team may tell you that it's unnecessary or unsafe. Please discuss this with them and find an experienced practitioner who can guide and advise you. The safety and efficacy data for ketosis in epileptic children is phenomenal.[19] There is solid safety data for ketosis in pediatric cancer as well.

While I recommend a high-fat, low-carbohydrate, and animal-based protein-rich diet, you can get to ketosis with different types of diets. Ketones don't just lower sugar; they also reduce inflammation, change your child's epigenetic expression, reduce angiogenesis, and rewire signaling pathways. Ketosis is a powerful tool.

You can do this.

CHAPTER 7

Evaluate General Integrative Therapies

As PARENTS, IT'S OUR JOB TO MAKE SURE OUR CHILDREN GET THE BEST care. When the best care is not available through conventional oncology—remember, it takes approximately seventeen years for research evidence to reach clinical practice—we have to find ways to fill in the gaps.[1] Nutrition and integrative therapies can sometimes help fill those gaps, especially when it comes to managing side effects and improving quality of life. This chapter will review different integrative therapies and their use in pediatric oncology. While there are many books that review these therapies for adults and many integrative practitioners who work with adult cancer patients in these modalities, few medical professionals are willing to touch the third rail of integrative therapies in pediatric cancer, even though there are many therapies that can benefit your child.

It is important that these therapies be used as part of an individualized protocol under the direction of an integrative practitioner. Without addressing your child's total terrain, none of these therapies will be as effective, and they may not be safe. For example, simply taking your child to an IV clinic for high-dose vitamin C without assessing their labs and current condition is not a safe or correct way to use this information. That said, there are a few very basic therapies that every child needs and that carry little to no risk. Beyond nutrition, these include: exceptional sleep, lots of time outdoors, movement, and emotional or spiritual care. These types of therapies are often an afterthought, tacked on at the end or forgotten about altogether, but I'm including them here at the beginning of the chapter to emphasize that, in many ways, these are, along with deep nutrition, among the most powerful tools at your disposal.

Basic Therapies for Every Child

The circadian rhythm is essential to healing. Sleep hygiene should be a primary concern for any parent who has a child diagnosed with cancer, especially since sleep disturbance is common during and after anticancer therapies.[2]

You know how this story goes: You get the devastating news of cancer. The stress keeps everyone in the house up. Your child starts inpatient treatment, and sleep goes entirely out the window. Now you have a child trying to sleep in an unfamiliar and uncomfortable place with IVs coming out of their body, machines beeping incessantly, and nurses visiting frequently. On top of that, anticancer therapy is very hard on the body. Quickly, sleep becomes something of the past—for your child, for you, often for the whole family.

However, your child's circadian rhythm and the quality of their sleep is essential to healing. Sleep-wake rhythm impairment is associated with more cancer-related fatigue in pediatric leukemia patients.[3] Circadian dysregulation is linked to poorer outcomes.

Simple interventions can support circadian health: Continue or create a bedtime routine that includes wind-down time with no electronics at least thirty minutes before bed. Your child might benefit from listening to a meditation or a bedtime story, or reading. Consider a warm bath with a drop of lavender essential oil. Full-spectrum hemp oil or chamomile tea can also be soothing. Keep the same bedtime every night, and allow your child to sleep in. Children going through treatment and healing post-treatment need extra rest. Protect your child's sleep and encourage naps.

Make the bedroom dark and cool. Take all electronics out of the room. (I realize this is not possible in a hospital.) If your child is inpatient, and if it is OK with nursing staff, cover the cardiac monitors with a towel or ask for them to be dimmed. Use cotton pajamas and sheets, preferably organic. Avoid polyesters and flame-retardant sheets and bedclothes.

Being outside is associated with many health benefits, including elevated mood, decreased risk of many disorders, healthier weight, fewer mental health issues, and better dietary decisions.[4] These benefits are especially important for children going through treatment—and their families. Place an emphasis in your family on time outside every day, as much as possible.

The practice of forest bathing refers to a walk in the woods without distraction.[5] It means taking in all the forest atmosphere, the sights and sounds and smells of the forest. Studies show that this can be particularly healing for a cancer patient. In one study, blood was sampled from subjects before and after forest bathing. The blood samples taken after forest bathing showed enhanced human NK cell activity and expression of anticancer proteins.[6]

Research also demonstrates that grounding—essentially walking barefoot in the grass, soil, or sand—can reduce pain, alter the number of circulating neutrophils and lymphocytes, reduce inflammation, and improve mood.[7] The science behind this is relatively simple: As bioelectrical organisms, humans carry a positive charge, which can build up in our bodies. The earth has a negative charge, so when we make contact through grounding, we discharge excess energy, which produces a healing effect. Swimming in oceans, lakes, or rivers is another method of grounding. You can even invest in a grounding mat for inside your home.

Movement is also an essential part of healing. It is very easy to stop moving during treatment. Your child feels sick, wants to sleep or lie around, and the family is overwhelmed and not focused on this part of therapy. However, we must remember that movement *is* therapy. Studies show that exercise training in children with cancer improves functional mobility.[8] Certain chemotherapy agents like vincristine can lead to nerve damage, and many kids stop walking altogether after this chemotherapy.[9] It is imperative to encourage daily movement in the hospital and when at home. Even better: Combine nature with movement, for two therapies in one. Take advantage of any inpatient physical therapy or services that encourage your child to move.

One of my biggest recommendations is rebounding, which is basically jumping on a trampoline. Get a large outdoor trampoline, and let the kids do the rest, with lots of time jumping and being outside. (Please install a net around the trampoline to avoid injuries.) Rebounding creates an increased gravitational load and positively stresses the cells in the body. This strengthens the musculoskeletal system, including the bones, muscles, and organs, as well as stimulating lymphatic circulation. A small indoor rebounder is useful in winter or bad weather.

Lastly, it's easy to get so caught up in conventional anticancer therapy, nutrition, and supplements that we forget the most important therapy: healing of the spirit. There are so many ways to incorporate emotional and spiritual healing for children. Consider what might work best for your child—it could be working with a therapist, guided meditation, breath work, music, the arts, and so much more. See chapter 12 for more on this aspect of healing.

Individualized Therapies

There are many integrative therapies. Don't attempt to layer all of these on your child. Instead, try to identify the right therapy for the right patient at the right time, with the help, of course, of an integrative practitioner. There is no protocol that works for every patient, not even those with the same type of cancer. The following list is a broad overview of therapies I have found to be most supportive and effective when used correctly.

To put it another way: The terrain-centric approach to healing starts with your child's story, beginning with your child's grandparents, their lives, where they lived, their illnesses, and their own personal journeys, and the same for you, your spouse, your child's siblings, and any other key member of your family. The story includes pregnancy and childbirth, as well as the histories of illnesses and medications, geographic location, and major life events. Why do we examine all these elements? It helps to identify things that may have contributed to the formation of cancer.

Refer back to the terrain assessment in chapter 4. Remember that this assessment helps to identify broken terrain in the child's life, which is then used to identify what may have contributed to the disease process. Layered on this assessment are genetic and epigenetic testing, biopsy results, and mutations. With all of these pieces, we can create a therapeutic plan that is individualized and supportive of your child. I don't mean a therapeutic plan for "this type of cancer" or "anticancer therapy" so much as I'm referring to what your child needs to heal, at a deeper level. Below you will find many therapies that can be supportive when they are used in a terrain-centric, individualized way. Many integrative practitioners can help you develop a plan that incorporates the most important lifestyle modifications, supplements, and integrative therapies layered with more conventional therapies. Let's start with a look at some supplements that I've found effective in supporting pediatric cancer.

Boswellia

Boswellia is a tree extract with a history of use in Ayurvedic medicine. It is anti-inflammatory and often used as an adjunct for cancer treatment. *Boswellia serrata*, also referred to as Indian frankincense, has been shown to be beneficial in brain-tumor-induced edema.[10] Studies also support the use of frankincense oil for cancer-related fatigue.[11] It is thought that boswellic acids may have an antiproliferative effect on tumors and inhibit the proliferation of tumor cells of the leukemia and glioblastoma subset.[12] *Boswellia* also helps stimulate programmed cell death. *Boswellia* can also be used in higher doses as an anti-inflammatory and can be supportive in weaning children off steroids. *Boswellia* can have possible interactions, especially with anticoagulants, so be sure to discuss with your integrative practitioner and oncology team. It can also have side effects, including digestive upset and mild blood thinning, so start with low doses and increase slowly. Dosages generally range from 500 to 4,500 milligrams daily, depending on the intended purpose and the weight of the child.

Cannabinoids

When my daughter was first diagnosed with cancer, we used cannabis oil secretly to help ease her nausea. Seven years later, there is little need for secrecy; the medical use of cannabis, even in children, is no longer taboo. I simply let my daughter's oncology team know that we are using a quality cannabis oil to help with chemotherapy-related nausea.

Medical cannabinoids are derived from either the cannabis plant or the hemp plant. The difference is the amount of the psychoactive substance delta-9-tetrahydrocannabinol (THC). In addition to THC, there are close to a hundred other therapeutic cannabinoids in the plant, one of the most well-known being CBD. Recently, the anticancer effects of other cannabinoids such as CBG have come to light.[13]

The human body actually has its own endocannabinoid system, which is sort of like the conductor of an orchestra, helping other systems—endocrine, cardiovascular, neurological—function and communicate better. Medical cannabinoids essentially enhance what the body already has the potential to do.

In my experience, medical cannabinoids can help you avoid having to use other, more risky, adjunct medications. For example, instead of pharmaceutical compounds for nausea, pain, sleep, or anxiety, medical cannabinoids can offer the same or similar benefits—and potentially, anticancer effects to boot. Studies support the use of medical cannabinoids for:

- balancing the immune system,[14]
- decreasing nausea and improving appetite,[15]
- supporting the ability to fall and stay asleep,[16]
- lowering the need for pain medication,[17]

- reducing inflammation,[18]
- decreasing and treating graft-versus-host disease,[19]
- potentially improving the efficacy of standard therapies,[20] and
- potential anticancer effect for certain cancers.[21]

Medical cannabinoid products include tinctures, gummies, suppositories, and topical products. I recommend oil tincture of full-spectrum hemp to start, as it has very little THC and will not cause patients to feel psychoactive effects. The dose depends on the goal. For example, it will be a different dose for nausea than for graft-versus-host disease. I recommend working with a practitioner experienced with medical cannabis.

In general, CBD products are safe even in high doses, whereas THC products may cause a high with mood changes and altered consciousness. Therefore, caution is essential in the pediatric population, and slow dose escalation is key. Check for possible interactions with other medications, and be mindful of the dose with elevated liver enzymes. Finally, know the law: Many places have legalized the use of medical cannabis–derived cannabinoids. For locations that have not, I recommend hemp-derived cannabinoids.

Quality is essential with medical cannabis products. With the booming industry of the past decade have come serious quality-control issues, including pesticide-sprayed plants, mold contamination during processing, and artificial colors and carcinogenic ingredients added to oils and gummy products. It is important to research any products you purchase for your child. Our family grows our own on land never touched by pesticides or herbicides. We then process this into oils and teas, which we sell under the name Twisted River Farms.

Vitamin C

While IV vitamin C is often associated with integrative oncology, oral vitamin C is also excellent for cancer prevention and reducing oxidative stress in cancer patients. Vitamin C promotes healthy immunity and helps treat and prevent infections. Humans are among the few mammals that do not make endogenous vitamin C, so we must get it from food or supplements.[22] Excessive intake of oral vitamin C can cause digestive upset, including diarrhea, which is why the high doses of vitamin C for cancer care are often administered through an IV. Vitamin C should be avoided on days of IV chemotherapy due to potential interaction. The dosage is typically 250 to 10,000 milligrams daily. I recommend liposomal for better absorption.

Vitamin D3

Vitamin D3 is a fat-soluble hormone found naturally in foods like salmon, sardines, butter, eggs, and cod liver oil, and is also formed in the skin when the skin is exposed to sunlight. Vitamin D can be tested through a blood test called 25-hydroxy vitamin D. Vitamin D deficiency is common in children with cancer and likely a contributing factor to the diagnosis.[23] Deficiency increases risk of relapse. A 2020 study found a significant correlation between vitamin D and prognosis.[24] In addition, low levels of vitamin D impact survivors of childhood cancer and contribute to their long-term health issues following treatment. Identifying vitamin D levels in childhood cancer survivors is critically important because optimizing the levels may help prevent secondary cancers and chronic disease.

Optimal levels are over 50 and closer to 100 nanomoles per liter for a pediatric patient. Typical dosage is 2,000 to 5,000 IU daily, depending on blood level. Vitamin D3 supplementation can also be used with other supplements to help prevent a cytokine storm and modulate the immune system. In this case it can be used in high doses for short bursts, especially during active treatment. I always recommend taking vitamin D with vitamin K2 to ensure that the calcium transported by the vitamin D is absorbed by the bones and is not accumulated and deposited in the arteries.

Fermented Wheat Germ Extract

Available as a powder or a tablet, fermented wheat germ extract (FWGE) is a nutritional supplement that blocks the glucose fuel supply of cancer. It also enhances immune function by increasing NK cell activity and causes cancer cell death, or apoptosis. Studies show FWGE reduces chemotherapy-induced febrile neutropenia in pediatric cancer patients.[25] Multiple studies support the use of FWGE as an adjunct to chemotherapy or radiation, as it decreases the progression of the disease, improves quality of life, and lessens the side effects of conventional treatment.[26] Some patients will experience digestive issues when using FWGE, and it should not be used in anyone with celiac disease or a gluten allergy. The dosage is typically based on weight, between 2 and 9 grams per day.

Fish Oil

Omega-3 fatty acids have become quite a controversial supplement! As you have likely heard, it has become challenging to procure quality fish—and therefore even more challenging to procure quality fish oil. Many integrative practitioners argue that all fish oil is rancid and prefer to source omega-3 fatty acids from plants instead. Unfortunately, omega-3 fatty acids from plants are much harder for our bodies to use, and DHA and EPA have more health benefits when they are from fish, according to many studies.[27]

Omega-3 fatty acids have natural anti-inflammatory effects that can limit cancer proliferation, initiate cancer cell death, and inhibit tumor blood supply.[28] Omega-3 fatty acids have also been shown to delay the progression of neuroblastoma in vivo and to be beneficial in counteracting malnutrition. A 2021 study concluded that omega-3 fatty acids exert various beneficial effects on the immune system, various metabolic pathways, and proliferation processes, and that DHA and EPA appear to be a relatively nontoxic form of supportive therapy.[29] Fish oil also helps improve the effectiveness of multiple chemotherapy agents, including doxorubicin, oxaliplatin, paclitaxel, and 5-FU.[30] Doses of up to 3,500 milligrams are considered safe in the pediatric cancer population.[31] Fish oil is generally well tolerated, except for digestive upset at higher doses. It also has an anticoagulant effect, so it's important to check for interactions with other medications.

Glutamine

Glutamine is an amino acid that is both produced by the body and supplied by food and supplements, and is needed for muscle growth and recovery. Glutamine is typically used to reduce chemotherapy side effects, but it is not considered an anticancer treatment and has some controversy associated with its use during active cancer. I use it to prevent mucositis and, in some situations, to protect the gut during chemotherapy.[32] Studies for safe doses for pediatric cancer patients have been conducted, and this therapy is becoming more accepted and used globally in conventional oncology situations.[33] I do not think glutamine should be supplemented long term for those with active cancer, but there is certainly a place for appropriate use. Dosage is typically 1 to 10 grams daily, depending on weight and indication.

Glutathione

Glutathione is a powerful antioxidant composed of three amino acids: cysteine, glutamic acid, and glycine. It is produced both endogenously and exogenously in fruits and vegetables. Vitamin C is a major enhancer of glutathione synthesis. Fat-soluble toxins and heavy metals are the main binding substrates for glutathione. Glutathione reduces oxidative stress–induced liver damage, which can occur from both chemotherapy and radiation.[34] Many anticancer therapies, including DCA, require and eat up a lot of glutathione. In fact, one argument against the use of acetaminophen is that it also depletes glutathione storage. In terms of labs, you can check total glutathione levels in blood or urine tests or find epigenetic glutathione SNPs through the Nutrition Genome test (see appendix A).

Glutathione is appropriate for all types of cancer, but caution should be exercised during chemotherapy and radiation. It is best used between treatments for recovery. (The exception would be if your child is on platinum-based chemotherapy.[35]) Intravenous, inhaled, or oral ingestion (liposomal) provide the best absorption. (It tastes like rotten eggs, so inhalation is often easiest for kids.) It can also be compounded into a nasal spray or patch. Dosage is based on the child's weight, but typically is 200 to 1,000 milligrams daily.

Helleborus

Helleborus niger is a perennial herb referred to as the Christmas rose. There are different types of *Helleborus*, and it is considered very safe, with no side effects other than potential allergy. It is typically used as adjunct therapy in the treatment of many cancers and related symptoms, including metastasis to the brain or lung, lymphoma, melanoma, leukemia, spinal and brain tumors, and graft-versus-host disease. Benefits include the inhibition of cancer cell growth, decreased inflammation, easier breathing for patients with lung issues, and decrease in tumor-related pain.[36] It is also used for mental resilience, anxiety, and depression. It is most commonly used to complement mistletoe therapy, but it can also be used by itself, most frequently via subcutaneous injection or inhalation.

Low-Dose Naltrexone (LDN)

Full-dose naltrexone is used in conventional medicine to treat drug and alcohol addiction. In micro doses, LDN is used off-label by practitioners all over the world for many different types of issues, including autoimmune diseases, multiple sclerosis, and generalized pain.[37] LDN is considered a therapeutic tool for all types of cancer. LDN causes increased cell death in certain cancers and potentially increases patient response to chemotherapy agents.[38] It can also reduce tumor growth by interfering with cell signaling as well as by modifying the immune system.

There are numerous studies supporting the use of LDN with various types of cancers. Dr. Bernard Bihari treated 450 cancer patients with LDN and reported that 270 of them had significant benefits from LDN, including a decrease in tumor size of at least 75 percent.[39] Penn State investigators Ian Zagon and his colleagues published evidence that a dose of 0.1 milligrams per kilogram in mice reduced neuroblastoma tumor incidence by 66 percent, slowed tumor growth by 98 percent, and increased survival by 36 percent over controls. LDN also supports the action of classic anticancer therapy like radiation and platinum chemotherapy drugs.[40] LDN can delay progression of disease and reduce risk of relapse. With its low side-effect profile, there is little reason *not* to be on LDN, other than if the patient is on narcotic pain medication, as it will block the pain medication effect. LDN is safe in children and used in pediatrics outside of oncology.

Dosing can start anywhere from 0.5 to 1.5 milligrams and increase slowly up to 4.5 milligrams. Children should be on their maximum dose daily for seven days before starting the on/off cycle, which consists of four days on and three days off. The days off should be before chemotherapy treatment (even though there are no known contraindications). Side effects can include disturbance in the form of vivid dreams that usually go away after a month, mild headache, or mild agitation; a few patients may have nausea or gastrointestinal effects. If a child has side effects, it's possible to start with an even lower dose of 0.25 milligrams and titrate slowly. LDN is available as liquid, tablet, topical, or in a rapid-dissolve form through a compounding pharmacy.

Melatonin

Melatonin is a hormone produced in the pineal gland, frequently also used in supplement form as a sleep aid. Melatonin is also excellent for the immune system, stimulating T cells and NK cells, lowering the toxicity of several chemotherapy agents, and reducing chemo side effects.[41] It also can reduce blood flow to a solid tumor and activate a tumor-suppressing gene.[42]

Melatonin is considered safe in pediatric cancer but should be avoided in high doses in leukemia. Dosage is typically between 3 and 60 milligrams, taken in the evening.

Medicinal Mushrooms

Turkey tail, chaga, reishi, maitaki, and shiitake are a few of the types of mushrooms with medicinal value. Medicinal mushrooms strengthen the immune system, help patients tolerate chemotherapy, and improve quality of life.[43] Unfortunately, most studies on medicinal mushrooms for cancer treatment have been on adults, so there is little data on pediatric patients, but most medicinal mushrooms are well tolerated. Dosage varies on type of mushroom. Work with a practitioner who is familiar with medicinal mushrooms and knowledgeable about how and when to incorporate them.

N-acetylcysteine

N-acetylcysteine (NAC) stimulates glutathione biosynthesis, promotes detoxification, and is one of the most important naturally occurring antioxidants. NAC is chemoprotective and helps mitigate nephrotoxicity from key chemotherapy agents.[44] In combination with vitamin E, it has been shown to reduce chemotherapy and radiation-related toxicities in pediatric acute lymphoblastic leukemia. NAC is also being studied for cisplatin-induced hearing loss and has been shown to reduce ototoxic damage in the 10,000 and 12,000 Hz frequencies.[45] Research also shows that NAC can inhibit cancer cell proliferation and tumor growth in glioblastoma therapy.[46]

Once used as a decongestant, NAC works as a supportive treatment in many cancers by starving the cancer cell. I also found through personal experience with my daughter that NAC can be used to treat a condition known as veno-occlusive disease (VOD), a potentially life-threatening side effect after a bone marrow transplant that starts with liver congestion from the toxicity of the transplant chemotherapy. In a small study of nine children with moderate to severe VOD, the use of intravenous NAC resulted in 100 percent cure from VOD within four to sixteen days.[47] NAC has also been studied to help prevent VOD. I kept my daughter on high doses of NAC through her second transplant, and we were able to avoid VOD entirely. NAC is typically well tolerated with dosage ranging from 500 milligrams to 6 grams per day, depending on its intended use and method of administration (oral or IV).

Quercetin

Quercetin is a flavonoid found in fruits and vegetables, including apples, dark-colored berries, grapes, olive oil, red wine, and onions, and is commonly used as a supplement for seasonal allergies. It is an antioxidant, antitumor agent, and anti-inflammatory, and also stimulates several detoxification enzymes to protect against environmental carcinogens. Studies show quercetin can be neuroprotective in pediatric diseases including central nervous system tumors and can also affect cancer cell death (apoptosis), proliferation, and chemoresistance of the osteosarcoma cells.[48] A 2014 study published in *Cancer Prevention Research* investigated the in vitro and in vivo multitarget effects of quercetin in leukemia, demonstrating that quercetin is an effective antitumor agent for hematologic malignancies.[49] Quercetin also shows significant antitumor effects in hepatocellular carcinoma.[50]

Quercetin is typically well tolerated but may interact with other medications, including but not limited to doxorubicin, cisplatin, anticoagulant medications, and quinolone antibiotics. Be sure there is no interaction between quercetin and your child's chemotherapy, as this is not uncommon. Dosage is based on weight and is usually around 500 to 2,000 milligrams daily.

Turmeric

A spice containing curcumin commonly used in Indian cooking, turmeric is also used as a nutritional supplement and has been recognized for centuries as a healing agent best known for its anti-inflammatory properties. It has been shown to induce cell death (apoptosis) in human neuroblastoma cells.[51] Its antitumor properties have also been studied in pediatric rhabdomyosarcoma, enhancing the effects of cytotoxic drugs, reducing migration, and increasing cancer cell death.[52] Cisplatin has also been shown to be more effective against pediatric epithelial liver tumors in combination with curcumin.[53] Turmeric also shows promise in brain tumors. Side effects are typically mild and include antiplatelet properties (thinning of the blood). Dosage (liposomal) is based on the child's weight, and is typically 500 to 8,000 milligrams daily.

Injection Therapies

Injection therapies may initially sound overwhelming and scary, but there are several reasons why certain injection therapies warrant consideration.

Some therapies, such as mistletoe, are only available as injections. In other cases, even when oral alternatives are available, intravenous administration is often more effective.

One of the challenges associated with IV therapy is the process of getting a needle inserted. Our children have already gone through a lot, and subjecting them to the stress of another poke is no fun for anyone. Often, the use of a central line is easier on kids than a poke, but not all children have a central line, port, or PICC line. Even if they do, some IV therapy clinics may refuse to access the port due to concerns about infection (and I don't recommend having just anyone access your child's central line either, even if they are willing to!).

It is crucial to be cautious when considering IV therapy clinics for your child's care. I recommend working with an integrative practice who has experience with pediatric patients. Moreover, it's important to note that not all IV therapies are created equal. Just as you can find poor-quality vitamins at corner pharmacies, you can also come across IV vitamin C that is made from corn. Therefore, it is essential to ensure that you receive high-quality IV therapies from a reputable source. But with well-trained IV staff and an integrative practice that specializes in cancer and pediatrics, the right IV therapy can make a significant difference for your child.

Mistletoe

Mistletoe therapy has been used for cancer care since the 1920s. It has an immunomodulatory effect on the immune system—neither overstimulating nor suppressing it, instead helping it work more efficiently. Mistletoe has been shown to induce cancer cell death (apoptosis) both directly by its cytotoxic effects and indirectly by supporting the immune cells.[54] It modulates the white blood cells, including NK cells, T helper cells, and T killer cells, all parts of our innate and adaptive immune system that are part of cancer surveillance.[55] Mistletoe can also limit cancer's ability to spread, and it can help stabilize and repair DNA.[56]

Mistletoe has particularly promising applications for pediatric osteosarcoma. A 2014 study compared the chemotherapy drug etoposide to mistletoe for patients in surgical remission after a second relapse and showed a five-year post-relapse disease-free survival rate of 55.6 percent in the mistletoe group and zero in the chemotherapy group.[57] In addition, mistletoe has a synergistic action in osteosarcoma when combined with etoposide.

The drawback of mistletoe is that, for it to be effective, it needs to be administered either subcutaneously or intravenously, usually one to three times a week. However, many children, once they get over the fear of the injection, do fine with this therapy, and many oncologists are open and curious and willing to explore mistletoe's therapeutic effects.

Mistletoe has a warming effect on the body, and the injection will produce a small (smaller than a silver-dollar-sized) red rash that should go away within twelve to twenty-four hours. There are different types of mistletoe, multiple ways to administer it, and no particular protocol based on weight or for the type of cancer. Avoid it if your child is being treated for a brain tumor or lung metastases with swelling. I recommend reading the book *Mistletoe and the Emerging Future of Integrative Oncology* by Steven Johnson and Nasha Winters and working with a mistletoe-therapy-trained practitioner.

High-Dose IV Vitamin C

High-dose IV vitamin C (IVC) is a popular therapy with a well-established safety profile that is increasingly accepted by conventional oncology. It is sometimes available in conventional oncology hospitals and clinics.[58] IVC is a powerful adjuvant treatment alongside many standard chemotherapies, helping to mitigate the toxic effects of chemo. IVC is a prooxidative, cytotoxic agent and anticancer epigenetic regulator and immunomodulator. (Epigenetic modulators can turn the expression of a mutation "on" or "off.") It is also a potent and highly effective antiviral. High-dose IVC can improve quality of life by improving appetite and platelet counts as well as helping with fatigue and pain. It can stabilize advanced cancers or arrest the growth and spread of tumors. Unfortunately, IV is the only effective way to administer high-dose vitamin C due to stomach upset. (Most patients can tolerate somewhere around 10 grams of vitamin C taken orally, and less for children.)

You need to check that your child does not have a G6Pd deficiency before using high-dose IVC. Don't have labs drawn in the twenty-four hours following high-dose IVC, as it will falsely show lower lab values for kidney function. Also, you should monitor monthly metabolic panels for creatinine (kidney function). Anyone with a history of kidney stones needs to be cautious with IVC use. Although rare, oxalate kidney stones can be aggravated by vitamin C. Hydration is key. Vitamin B6 and magnesium may help reduce oxalate in the urine as well. Naturally, always consult with a trained practitioner.

High-dose IVC should be given at least two times per week for eight to twelve weeks. It should also never be stopped abruptly but should be slowly weaned over time. For example, you might administer it twice per week for three to six months, reduce it to once per week for another three to six months, then once every other week, and then once per month. A minimum of twenty-four infusions are needed to determine if it is an effective therapy for a given patient.

While adult high-dose IVC has particular dosing, in a child it is based on body weight at 0.4 to 1.4 grams per kilogram and is generally not administered with glutathione or other nutrients or antioxidants on the same day.[59] Some patients may experience nausea, headache, or fatigue for a day or two after an infusion. High-dose IVC is considered very safe when administered by a qualified practitioner and in a sterile environment.

Dichloroacetate (DCA)

Dichloroacetate (DCA) is a small molecule that has historically been used to treat a metabolic disorder called lactic acidosis. It works by inhibiting lactate formation and switches the cell metabolism to mitochondrial energy metabolism. Mitochondria regulate many processes that are known to be altered in cancer cells including metabolism. The metabolic approach to cancer looks to mitochondrial metabolism as a target for cancer therapy—and theorizes that it is the damage of our mitochondria that leads to the development of cancer. DCA is also able to cause cancer cell death due to the metabolic differences between most cancer cells and normal cells, and this weakens the cancer cell. It has also been shown to make platinum chemotherapies more effective.[60]

DCA can be administered orally or by IV. The IV DCA is more effective, but sometimes oral administration is preferable for children. Due to its mechanism, the patient should be in a state of therapeutic ketosis for DCA treatment to be most effective. When administered by an experienced practitioner, it can be safe, with reversible side effects. (Self-limited neuropathy or dizziness is not uncommon, and DCA is contraindicated if your child already experiences neuropathy.) The relevant labs are CBC and CMP to assess any potential rare side effects such as elevation of liver enzymes or lower platelets.

While it can be used for all types of cancer, DCA has been shown to be particularly effective for glioblastoma.[61] DCA can be given as a combination of IV and oral administration—IV twice per week combined with oral administration four times per week. Alternatively, it can be administered entirely orally or inhaled four to five times per week. Regardless of the administration method, DCA should always be used with Poly MVA (but not necessarily the other way around) to help prevent the tingling and neuropathy one may experience with DCA.

Poly MVA

Poly MVA is a supplement that contains minerals, B-complex vitamins, palladium, amino acids, alpha-lipoic acid, molybdenum, rhodium, ruthenium, thiamine, riboflavin, cyanocobalamin, N-acetylcysteine, and N-formylmethionine. (The palladium allows the alpha-lipoic acid to reach cells in the body.) It is a complex polymer molecule that supports mitochondrial energy production and can help with fatigue. In studies, Poly MVA has been shown to enhance the antitumor effect of radiation, protect against DNA damage in peripheral blood, and protect against radiation-induced reduction of platelet count.[62] Poly MVA can be an excellent supplement for neuropathy.

Poly MVA can be taken orally or administered via intravenous infusion, which takes approximately thirty to forty-five minutes. Intravenous infusions have been found to be safe and tolerable with minimal side effects, though I tend to prefer oral administration for children. Some patients will experience a marked increase in energy.

Other Therapies

In addition to the individualized therapies and the injection therapies I've already covered, there are various other therapies that can be useful. Some of these therapies, like essential oils, can be a soothing adjuvant therapy for symptom management, but are not necessary if your child doesn't enjoy them. It is important to know that there is such a thing as essential oil toxicity, so while oils are not invasive, their effects can be powerful, both for good and for bad. Other therapies, like hyperbaric oxygen chamber usage, can, in some cases, be relevant to the outcome of the disease but *must* be used under the guidance of a knowledgeable practitioner.

I share these therapies with you to give you information on what is available, not to overwhelm you with options. It is always best to introduce one new therapy at a time, so you can note the effect. It is better to focus on sustainably using the key therapies for your child's specific disease than to throw the kitchen sink at it. More is not always better.

Pulsed Electromagnetic Field (PEMF) Mat

A PEMF mat heats up and converts electricity into infrared rays. It penetrates the body up to eight inches, stimulating the healing and regeneration of nerves and muscle tissue. Studies support the use of a PEMF mat for reducing inflammation, managing acute and chronic pain, improving sleep, promoting circulation, and fostering a sense of well-being.[63] I often turn to these devices for localized pain or inflammation relief. We used a Biomat with Zuza in the hospital and for post conventional cancer therapy during her healing and while she was meditating. To avoid burns, don't use these devices on the head or sensitive skin. Popular brands include Biomat and Bemer (see appendix D for details).

Essential Oils

Essential oils are concentrated plant extracts. Practitioners use them in various ways, such as aromatherapy and massage. Many essential oils have been studied for their use on cancer patients; the most well-known are lavender for nausea and peppermint for headache. It is important to remember that essential oils are potent and should be used with caution.

Homeopathy

Homeopathy uses very diluted substances to provoke the body's own healing systems to higher function. The practice of homeopathy emerged in the nineteenth century and was used frequently at that time, often more successfully than allopathy. In fact, in the 1918 influenza epidemic, homeopathic hospitals reported a statistically significant higher success rate than allopathic hospitals.[64] In 1910, however, the American Medical Association, with the aid of the pharmaceutical industry, drafted a congressional report that favored funding for allopathic medical schools rather than homeopathic schools, leading to the dropping off of homeopathic training and education.[65] I have not been trained in homeopathy and therefore rarely use these therapies myself. I do, however, encourage working with homeopaths to complement care.

Hyperbaric Oxygen Therapy (HBOT)

Hyperbaric therapy is known for treating decompression sickness and has evolved over time for use with many other conditions, including cancer care.

Hyperbaric oxygen therapy (HBOT) works by increasing the amount of oxygen in the body, so more is absorbed by the lungs and enters the bloodstream. This stimulates many healing processes, including stem cell production and fighting infections.

However, HBOT can also stimulate the growth of new blood vessels, prompting the growth of cancer as well, so if there is active disease, it is essential that a patient be in a therapeutic ketosis during HBOT. It is contraindicated in cases of pneumothorax, and care should be taken to avoid pain or trauma to the ear.

I recommend considering HBOT in conjunction with Poly MVA/DCA. It has also been shown to be effective in treating late radiation tissue injury in patients. Studies support its use for brain tumors, specifically gliomas when used before and after radiation treatment. Patients who used HBOT with radiation had a better prognosis than when radiation was used alone. HBOT may improve the ability of radiotherapy to kill hypoxic cancer cells and therefore the administration of radiotherapy while breathing hyperbaric oxygen can reduce mortality and recurrence.[66] If radiotherapy is part of your child's treatment plan, I suggest exploring HBOT with the oncology team. HBOT can also be a good post-chemotherapy recovery tool. The protocol is often one dive per week with at least 1.3 ATA, but this is highly dependent on the recommendations of your integrative oncology practitioner.

Ozone

Ozone gas is a form of oxygen therapy. Ozone has one extra molecule (O_3) and is like oxygen on steroids. O_3 has been shown to make chemotherapy and radiation more effective and reduce side effects.[67] It can also significantly reduce fatigue—up to 70 percent![68] Ozone has also been shown to reduce the intestinal tissue injury from methotrexate, a common pediatric chemotherapy.[69] Ozone is a wonderful adjunct to chemotherapy and radiation.

O_3 can be applied topically, rectally, nasally, aurally, vaginally, and intravenously. IV O_3 should only be administered by a trained professional. I prefer rectal ozone for the pediatric cancer patient, as it is less invasive than intravenous; this method also works well for postconventional gut-healing treatment. It is important to conduct a lab test for G6PD deficiency, in which case IV ozone is contraindicated. IV and hyperbaric ozone should also be avoided in the case of a heparin allergy.

Infrared Sauna

Sauna is an excellent therapy for detoxification, reducing inflammation, managing pain, and improving mood. In many cancers, some type of environmental toxicity (such as glyphosate) contributed to the diagnoses; glyphosate, other fat-soluble toxins, heavy metals, and estrogen dominance all can be reduced with the use of sauna. Even if your child did not have any toxicities that contributed to their diagnosis, they will have toxicities after they are done with chemotherapy.

A 2022 study published in the *Journal of Cancer Science and Therapy* found that after thirty days of infrared sauna treatment at temperatures as low as 77°F (25°C), tumor-infected mice had reductions of cancerous masses up to 86 percent.[70] A Japanese study published in *Internal Medicine* found that patients with chronic pain experienced pain-level reduction of up to 70 percent with just one session of infrared sauna.[71]

The protocol will depend on the reason for use but will generally range from two to six days per week for twenty to sixty minutes each time. The key with kids is to go slow. Start with a low temperature and five to ten minutes the first week and slowly increase time and temperature until you get to a comfortable space where the child is sweating for at least ten minutes. For most children, this will take at least twenty minutes with a temperature of at least 120°F (49°C). Be aware that sauna treatment can make patients dizzy or lightheaded. Keep your child hydrated and—again—go slowly. Exercise additional caution with young children and children with shunts or ports or feeding tubes. Check with the manufacturer of the child's device (that is, the shunt, port, or feeding tube) regarding the safety of that device in an infrared sauna.

Hyperthermia

Hyperthermia is a type of treatment in which the body tissue is heated up, either locally or systemically, to help damage and kill cancer cells and while preserving healthy cells. Most forms of hyperthermia that are effective are not approved in the United States. There is whole-body hyperthermia and localized hyperthermia, both of which, depending on the cancer, can be effective. Cancer cells are more sensitive to heat damage than healthy cells. A temperature of 108°F (42°C) must be reached for the therapy to be effective. Although there are numerous clinics in Europe and Mexico that perform this therapy, they do not accept children. This is unfortunate—tuck this one away for future use if the regulatory situation changes.

Red Light Therapy

Red light therapy supports circadian rhythm health and reduces inflammation, and it can be especially beneficial during inpatient stays.[72] Use the red light in the morning and evening to help your child regulate their sleep patterns and circadian rhythm. Red light therapy has been shown to reduce cancer-related side effects like insomnia, depression, and cognitive impairments.[73] Light therapy can also be used to heal skin after radiation. In one study, light therapy accelerated healing of skin damage from radiation therapy by up to 50 percent.[74] Red light therapy is typically used once or twice a day for about ten minutes. It should be avoided if your child is taking photosensitive medications.

Photodynamic therapy is another form of light therapy. This approach to cancer treatment relies on the administration of a photosensitizer followed by tumor illumination to generate oxidative stress and activate cell death mechanisms. Currently, intravenously photodynamic therapy can only be found outside of the United States or at select integrative oncology practices. It is not an FDA-approved therapy in the United States at the time of this writing.

Reiki

Reiki is an energy therapy in which a Reiki practitioner directs healing energy to a specific part of the body or through the entire body. It is considered safe for all ages. Studies show that Reiki is helpful in improving well-being, sleep quality, pain relief, and reducing anxiety and fatigue.[75]

———

The integrative therapies discussed here are ones I have personal and professional experience with and, in my estimation, are the safest and most effective for children with cancer. There are many other popular (but often ineffective) therapies that I chose not to include. As always, the key is to use your best judgment, consult with your child's oncology team, and always work with an experienced practitioner.

Additionally, continually assessing your child is key to understanding if a chosen therapy is effective and worthwhile for your individual child. Now that you have a broad general understanding of some integrative therapies, let's discuss some targeted therapies for certain types of pediatric cancer.

CHAPTER 8

Evaluate Cancer-Specific Integrative Therapies

EVERY PATIENT IS DIFFERENT AND HAS A DIFFERENT COMBINATION OF factors that led to the development of cancer. Although it's impossible to completely individualize care in a book, in this chapter I'll offer examples of therapies that I have seen to be effective with certain types of cancers. Truthfully, I debated whether or not to include this chapter, because I believe so strongly that treatment must be individualized and I do not want to suggest otherwise. On the other hand, it didn't feel right to me to withhold information that I could imagine being useful to a parent supporting their child with cancer. That being said, please do not use the information in this chapter as a protocol for your child; use it instead as a starting point for possibilities to consider and questions to ask.

Regrettably, I cannot cover every diagnosis. In this chapter, I focus on the most common pediatric cancers: leukemia, brain and spinal cord tumors, neuroblastoma, Wilms tumor, lymphoma (both Hodgkin and non-Hodgkin), rhabdomyosarcoma, bone cancer (including osteosarcoma and Ewing sarcoma), and adrenocortical carcinoma. At the end of the chapter, I'll cover therapies to specifically support hematopoietic stem cell transplantation (bone marrow transplants), as well as best practices to support your child in clinical trials.

Leukemia

Leukemia is the most common cancer among children. There are different types of leukemia, the most common being acute lymphoblastic leukemia (ALL). Less common and often more aggressive is acute myeloid leukemia (AML). Treatment of ALL is difficult because it is prolonged and includes not only chemotherapy but also steroids. AML treatment is shorter, if effective, but very toxic and often requires a bone marrow transplant.

Most leukemias are the result of a toxic chemical exposure, either in the mother or after the child is born.[1] I find a lot of glyphosate toxicity in leukemia patients. ALL is also associated with a compromised microbiome due to lack of exposure to diverse bacteria.[2] It has a complete remission rate of 90 percent; within five years up to 10 percent of children relapse. Relapse often leads to a possibility of radiation, CAR-T therapy, or a bone marrow transplant.

AML often needs chemotherapy and reinforcement with a bone marrow transplant. The five-year survival of children diagnosed with AML is up to 65 percent, but many relapse or are diagnosed with secondary cancers even outside of the five-year survival window.

When my daughter was diagnosed with AML, why didn't I just treat her "naturally"? I get this question a lot, so I want to answer it here: I have supported her with many integrative therapies, and it has made all the difference, but my experience is that acute pediatric leukemia requires chemotherapy.

In leukemia, the broken terrain often includes the microbiome, toxicity, and nutrition. Hematological malignancies respond well to carbohydrate restriction. During active AML treatment, therapeutic ketosis can help protect healthy cells and reduce side effects. For children with ALL, ketosis is recommended for the beginning of treatment and intermittently during IV chemo infusions. Once the child is out of the initial phase of treatment and moves onto a maintenance protocol, a low-carbohydrate, nutrient-dense diet should be followed (Level 1 Nutrition; see chapter 6). A 2021 study has shown that long-chain fatty acids are beneficial specifically for AML, which is part of why we eat lots of avocados in our family (at least ½ or a full avocado per day, plus pure, organic avocado oil).[3]

Melatonin and astragalus are contraindicated in all acute leukemias, as they can stimulate cancer growth. Important labs include the trifecta (CRP-HS, LDH, sed rate; see chapter 3). The neutrophil to lymphocyte ratio is important to monitor during treatment and remission. A bone marrow biopsy will confirm diagnosis or remission.

Possible Supplements

- Vitamin D3 with vitamin K2
- Full-spectrum CBD oil (and THC if legal)
- Low-dose naltrexone
- Fish oil
- Quercetin

- Poly MVA
- Turmeric
- Milk thistle
- Vitamin A

Possible IV or Injection Therapies

- Mistletoe A or P
- *Helleborus* D12 or D6
- Poly MVA/DCA protocol
- High-dose IVC

Brain and Spinal Cord Tumors

Brain and spinal cord tumors are the second most common cancer in children and the most common solid tumor affecting children. Approximately 20 percent of all pediatric cancers start in the brain, and nearly 5,000 new brain and spinal cord tumors are diagnosed in children each year.[4] There are many malignant kinds, the most aggressive being astrocytoma, glioblastoma, and diffuse intrinsic pontine glioma, which is highly aggressive and difficult to treat. Depending on the type of tumor, conventional treatment can include surgery, radiation, and potentially chemotherapy. Again, depending on the type of tumor, the five-year survival rate is 40 to 80 percent. Emerging research in mouse models is demonstrating success by interrupting metabolic pathways associated with glucose and glutamine and an epigenetic pathway associated with H3.3K27M mutations.[5]

Therapeutic ketosis when treating central nervous system tumors is important, as is the use of MCT oil and organic food and contaminant-free water. Intermittent fasting will help the child stay in ketosis. This is a type of tumor that may need continued therapeutic ketosis to keep the cancer from progressing. Potassium-rich foods are helpful to counteract the mood swings and pain from dexamethasone (steroids). The broken terrain is often related to EMF exposure and environmental toxins.

Mistletoe has been shown to have cytotoxic and apoptotic effects on medulloblastoma cancer cells.[6] (Medulloblastoma accounts for more than 20 percent of pediatric brain tumors.[7])

Glioblastoma has the highest mortality rate among primary brain tumors and continues to be poorly managed by conventional oncology. There are multiple published reports of patients refusing standard of care treatment other than surgery (and a ketogenic diet), who remain alive and without disease progression.[8] Specifically with glioma, a ketogenic diet is an important therapeutic tool. The most frustrating part of this therapy is that most patients need to stay on this type of diet long term. (This can be especially hard for tweens, in my experience.) With this type of cancer, getting the child into ketosis should be a primary goal. Most patients with glioma and brain tumors have radiation as part of their treatment protocol, however, and studies have shown that ketones may act as a radio sensitizing agent.[9] Hyperbaric oxygen therapy (two times per week) while in ketosis, as well as CBD oil and cannabis, can be effective.[10] Trifecta labs (CRP-HS, LDH, sed rate) are not as sensitive to central nervous system tumors.

Possible Supplements

- MCT oil
- *Boswellia* (this can reduce need for steroids)
- Oxaloacetate
- Oral or nebulized DCA
- Poly MVA
- Berberine
- Vitamin A
- Exogenous ketones
- Turmeric
- Low-dose naltrexone
- Vitamin D3
- Full-spectrum CBD
- Lion's mane
- Quercetin
- Valganciclovir
- Integrative Therapeutics Cortisol Manager (for symptoms of dexamethasone, or steroids)

Possible IV or Injection Therapies

- Poly MVA/DCA protocol
- *Helleborus* subcutaneous injection
- Mistletoe, with caution

Neuroblastoma

Neuroblastoma starts in early forms of nerve cells and almost always occurs in infants and young children. Like other pediatric-only cancers, there is very little information about the integrative support of neuroblastoma. It accounts for approximately 6 percent of all pediatric cancers and approximately 800 new cases are diagnosed each year.[11] Ninety percent of these cases are in children under the age of five. Prognosis predictions depend highly on the risk. The common broken terrain is EMF and toxic exposure.

Recently, studies have shown that this type of cancer responds well to a ketogenic diet, which can help make the neuroblastoma therapy more effective by inhibiting the viability of neuroblastoma cells.[12] A 2015 study shows that both a ketogenic diet and DCA can be used as therapeutic strategies in neuroblastoma.[13] I recommend using a ketogenic diet at minimum through treatment and ideally for a few years after, during the highest risk of relapse. Hyperbaric therapy can be used in combination with ketosis, and all families with neuroblastoma patients should reduce EMF exposure in the home.

Possible Supplements

- Vitamin D3
- MCT oil
- Vitamin A
- Oral or nebulized DCA
- Poly MVA
- Quercetin
- *Boswellia*
- Low-dose naltrexone
- *Taraxacum officinale* (dandelion)

Possible IV and Injection Therapies

- Poly MVA/DCA protocol

Wilms Tumor

Wilms tumor is a cancer of the kidney, most common in children ages three to four, and less likely to be diagnosed after the age of five. It most often occurs in one kidney, and prognosis is good. While this is a highly treatable cancer, there are kids who relapse, and even the standard treatment can be very toxic to such a young child. The common broken terrain includes nutrition, the microbiome, and emotional experiences. Wilms tumor cells demonstrate high glucose uptake. Targeting the Warburg effect by significantly reducing glucose and insulin, increasing ketone bodies, and reducing inflammation may be a promising therapeutic strategy against Wilms tumor.[14] I recommend a therapeutic ketogenic diet through conventional oncology treatment and ideally for a year beyond before changing to a low-carbohydrate, nutrient-dense diet. Hyperbaric oxygen during ketosis can also be beneficial.

Possible Supplements

- Oral or nebulized DCA
- Poly MVA
- MCT oil
- Full-spectrum CBD
  (and THC if legal)
- Vitamin D3
- Vitamin A
- Quercetin
- Turmeric
- Low-dose naltrexone

IV/Injection Therapies

- High-dose IVC
- Poly MVA/DCA protocol
- Mistletoe
- IV quercetin

Lymphoma

Lymphoma, both Hodgkin and non-Hodgkin, is found in the lymphoid tissue and shares many similarities with leukemia. About 12 percent of all cancers in kids are non-Hodgkin lymphomas.[15] The five-year survival rate is 97 percent for Hodgkin and 90 percent for non-Hodgkin. Administration of antibiotics more than ten times during childhood correlates with an 80 percent increased risk of developing non-Hodgkin lymphoma.[16] The use of steroids, such as cortisone, more than fifteen times multiplies the risk of non-Hodgkin lymphoma by 268 times.[17] Treatment consists of chemotherapy and radiation and the repeated use of highly potent drugs, often provoking secondary cancers. Mistletoe, specifically *Viscum album*, can be curative for certain types of lymphomas. The common broken terrain includes the microbiome; toxic exposure including, but not limited to, glyphosate and other pesticides; and poor nutrition, specifically refined and processed sugars and grains. Due to the intensity of treatment, I recommend therapeutic ketosis with the continuation of a low-carbohydrate, nutrient-dense diet after remission.

Possible Supplements

- Vitamin D3 with vitamin K2
- Full-spectrum CBD (and THC if legal)
- Low-dose naltrexone
- Fish oil
- Quercetin
- Poly MVA
- Turmeric

Possible IV and Injection Therapies

- Mistletoe
- High-dose IVC
- Poly MVA/DCA protocol

Rhabdomyosarcoma

There are approximately 500 new cases of rhabdomyosarcoma each year, with most diagnoses among children and teenagers.[18] It accounts for approximately 3 percent of pediatric cancer diagnoses.[19] Although relapses are common, there is still a five-year 70 percent survival rate. Genetic factors can contribute to the disease, including TP53 mutations and other rare syndromes. In vivo and in vitro studies that show *Viscum* (mistletoe) can effectively reduce tumor volume, and that *Viscum album* can support long-term survival.[20]

Children undergoing rhabdomyosarcoma treatment should be in ketosis. The chemotherapy drugs used are intense, and ketosis helps protect the healthy cells and improve treatment efficacy. In addition to treatment, a nutrient-dense, low-carbohydrate diet (Level 1 Nutrition) is key for healing.

Possible Supplements

- Oral or nebulized DCA
- Poly MVA
- MCT oil
- Full-spectrum CBD (and THC if legal)
- Vitamin D3
- Vitamin A
- *Boswellia*
- Quercetin
- Low-dose naltrexone

Possible IV and Injection Therapies

- High-dose IVC (+/− artesunate)
- Poly MVA/DCA protocol
- Mistletoe

Bone Cancer (Osteosarcoma and Ewing Sarcoma)

Osteosarcoma is a tumor that occurs in the bone, usually near the growth plate around the knee, arms, legs, or pelvis. Ewing sarcoma forms on bone or surrounding tissue. Treatment usually involves surgery and intense chemotherapy. Common broken terrain is toxin exposure and stress/emotional health. I recommend therapeutic ketosis through the intense chemotherapy treatment and then transitioning to Foundation Nutrition.

Mistletoe therapy can be very valuable for osteosarcoma. A randomized study on post-relapse disease compared mistletoe with oral etoposide, a chemotherapy that has multiple side effects and late effects. The five-year post-relapse, disease-free survival rate for this cancer is around 20 percent after a second recurrence. In the study, ten patients received oral etoposide for three weeks, every twenty-eight days for six months. In the other group, nine patients received subcutaneous *Viscum* (mistletoe) therapy three times per week for a year. The white blood cell counts of those treated with the chemotherapy drug etoposide showed a decrease in T cells. Those treated showed an increase in the CD3, CD4, and NK cells. The ten-year post-relapse, disease-free survival rate was 55.5 percent in the mistletoe group. In the oral etoposide group, it was zero.[21] Previous studies have shown that mistletoe has a synergistic effect with etoposide in osteosarcomas.[22]

Potential Supplements

- Oral or nebulized DCA
- Poly MVA
- Full-spectrum CBD (and THC if legal)
- Vitamin D3
- Vitamin A
- *Boswellia*
- Quercetin
- Low-dose naltrexone

Possible IV and Injection Therapies

- High-dose IVC
- Poly MVA/DCA protocol
- Mistletoe

Adrenocortical Carcinoma

Adrenocortical carcinoma is when malignant cells form in the outer layer of the adrenal gland.[23] It is extremely rare, seen in about 0.2 percent of pediatric cancers. Having the TP53 gene increases that risk of adrenocortical carcinoma. Surgery and chemotherapy are the treatment options, and immunotherapy is under investigation as a treatment option. The common broken terrain might include toxic exposure, damage to the microbiome, and emotional trauma. In addition to taking a child through conventional treatment in ketosis, I have had good experience with patients staying in ketosis for one to two years following treatment.

Possible Supplements

- Poly MVA
- Full-spectrum CBD (and THC if legal)
- Vitamin D3
- Vitamin A
- Quercetin
- Low-dose naltrexone

Possible IV and Injection Therapies

- High-dose IVC
- Mistletoe

Hematopoietic Stem Cell Transplantation (Bone Marrow Transplants)

Some pediatric cancer patients undergo the transplantation of hematopoietic stem cells (also referred to as a stem cell or bone marrow transplant), usually derived from bone marrow, peripheral blood, or umbilical cord blood, in order to produce additional normal blood cells. Transplants can be autologous, in which the patient donates their own stem cells, or allogeneic, in which someone else donates them. Autologous transplants are commonly used in neuroblastoma. Allogeneic transplants are also used in blood cancers like ALL and AML.

While potentially lifesaving, transplants can lead to many complications and side effects. The required chemotherapy or radiation is so toxic that it is imperative for patients to focus on healing their body and preventing potential late effects. The best way to go through transplant is in ketosis and to stay in ketosis for weeks to months afterward, as the body adapts to its new immune system. Ideally, the patient achieves ketosis at least one week before the transplant to prepare the body and ensure deep ketosis throughout the transplant process. Therapeutic ketosis is especially important during infusion days or what is referred to as conditioning—the chemotherapy/radiation protocol used to prepare the current bone marrow for new stem cells.

I highly encourage patients to remain in a deep therapeutic ketosis the entire inpatient stay. The key to staying in ketosis through transplant is careful planning of food packing and delivery to the hospital. Most hospitals do not serve food that would keep a child in ketosis (or that is even remotely nutritious), so you must bring your own.

My daughter, Zuza, has undergone multiple transplants. I used the therapies below and kept her in deep ketosis with an NG tube the first time and a G tube the second time. Both times she did extremely well mitigating side effects, including mucositis, which is extraordinarily painful. Up to 98 percent of patients get severe oral mucositis with myeloablative regiments, and up to 75 percent of patients get mucositis with reduced intensity regiments such as chemotherapy and radiation. I have applied the same protocol for many other adult and pediatric patients, who have achieved the same results. Reducing the risk of mucositis also reduces the need for narcotics, results in less constipation, decreases the risk of falls, and reduces the risk of secondary infections, resulting in fewer complications, fewer prolonged hospital stays, and decreased need for antibiotics. Keeping a patient in ketosis also results in better energy and well-being before, during, and after the transplant.

As I've mentioned already, you'll want to avoid dextrose in IV fluids; request normal saline instead. You'll also want to avoid steroids when possible, because they'll pull your child out of ketosis. If you must use steroids, add additional exogenous ketones to your child's protocol. Also steer clear of acetaminophen when possible, as well as unnecessary proton-pump inhibitors. A transplant is a complicated and risky procedure. It is essential that you communicate fully and clearly with your child's oncology team and work closely with an experienced integrative practitioner.

Possible Supplements

- Full-spectrum CBD in 50 to 200 milligram doses to prevent graft-versus-host disease
- Vitamin D3
- Vitamin A
- Quercetin (at least six hours before or after chemotherapy infusions)
- N-acetylcysteine
- Omega-3s
- Gastrazyme (from Biotics Research)
- L-glutamine, 3 to 5 grams starting day +1

Trials

If your child enters a clinical trial, you must work with a metabolically trained practitioner who understands the trial so you can support your child in the best way possible. Most trials are very strict about incorporating treatments other than the trial drug, so make sure you understand the trial, the drug, and its potential side effects. Nutrition can always be used to support your child. Please work with a trained practitioner.

Palliative Care

The issue of palliative care has been raised many times for our family, most recently after Zuza's second bone marrow transplant. Zuza got very upset at the idea of not pursuing a cure even if it meant more toxic therapies. If you are reading this book, you may eventually find yourself in this heartbreaking situation. Every patient is different, and all families are different, and so it is a very individual decision—there is no general advice that can be given and no "right" answer.

If your child is young and not capable of making this decision, you must make it for them. If your child is old enough, then they need to be part of the decision of continuing or ending treatment. For most cancers, ending conventional treatment does not necessarily mean you are choosing palliative care but instead means you will be focusing on less toxic therapies that can sometimes be equally effective. The quality of your child's life is more important than the quantity of their days. These are impossible decisions and impossible feelings. They are also decisions that you as a family can take time to make.

One way forward is to return to the concept of the broken terrain that may have contributed to your child's diagnoses in the first place and approach their palliative care by healing that aspect of their life while at the same time supporting any conventional anticancer therapy. A treatment plan becomes very individualized when you use a patient's terrain alongside the details of their cancer and treatment. This is when a truly individualized plan can be formed.

CHAPTER 9

Manage Side Effects

PEDIATRIC CANCER TREATMENT IS EXTREMELY TOXIC AND, FOR MOST types of cancer, has not improved in decades. There is no pediatric cancer treatment that does not produce either side effects or late effects or both. Side effects are an immediate or slightly delayed reaction to surgery, chemotherapy, radiation, or immunotherapy. Late effects start years after conventional cancer treatment and include secondary cancers, heart problems, lung problems, and emotional and cognitive issues. To combat side effects, oncologists dose additional pharmaceutical medications; they rarely address measures to prevent late effects.

For this reason, integrative medicine has a lot to offer for managing the side effects and late effects of conventional cancer care. In this chapter, I'll cover common side effects and effective methods for mitigating them. I'll start broadly, with common side effects from surgery, radiation, and chemotherapy, and then break things down further into different subclasses of chemotherapy.

Surgery

Surgery is used to both diagnose and treat cancer. Surgery for diagnosis involves removing a tissue sample (and possibly surrounding lymph nodes) and using a pathology lab to assess if cancer is present and, if so, what type it is. Surgery is also used to remove cancer for both curative and debulking options. It is considered the least toxic of all conventional cancer therapies.

These are my recommendations for preparing for surgery.

- For one month prior to surgery, give your child 1 to 4 tablespoons of fresh ground flaxseed daily to reduce tumor aggressiveness.
- For one week prior to surgery, avoid any herbs and supplements that can interact with sedatives and anesthetics.

- For three days prior to surgery, avoid any medications that can cause bleeding, such as ginger, turmeric, green tea, coenzyme Q10, fish oil, or high-dose vitamin C.
- The day before surgery, give your child 6C potency homeopathic hypericum and arnica to treat nerve injury and heal inflammation.
- Prior to surgery, feed your child low-carbohydrate, nutrient-dense food.

Immediately after surgery, give your child vitamin C, zinc citrate, and vitamin A with quality protein powder to support wound healing, along with methylated B-complex vitamins (with B5) and a multitrace mineral complex. Have your child begin to move around as soon as possible. Use bromelain to reduce pain and reduce risk of blood clots and edema. Control post-surgery inflammation with turmeric and grape-seed extract. Give your child IV nutrients similar to a Myers' IV. (Myers' IV is a standard nutrient IV formulated by the late John Myers, MD, with a good balance of vitamins and minerals; most nutritional IVs are variations of Myers' IV.)

Immunotherapy

Immunotherapy is a treatment intended to support the patient's own immune system in fighting cancer and infection. It includes monoclonal antibodies, cytokines, and treatment vaccines and can be used in combination with other treatments or alone. While immunotherapy sounds like it would be less toxic than chemotherapy, it can have just as many, if not more, devastating results on our organs. Different types of immunotherapy work in different ways. Some help the immune system stop the growth of cancers, while others help the immune system stop the cancer from spreading. At the time of this writing, immunotherapy is mostly used in off-study and experimental situations for different types of pediatric cancers.

Some of the drugs in this class include Keytruda, Raptiva, and Remicade (there are many more but these are the ones currently most common in pediatric cancer treatment). Side effects can include fever, chills, weakness, headache, nausea, vomiting, diarrhea, low blood pressure, rash, and bleeding.

Radiation

Radiation therapy, which has been used for cancer since the 1800s, works by administering photons or particles to tissue, whereby negatively charged molecules known as free radicals are formed. These free radicals damage both cancer cells and healthy cells. There is external radiation therapy and internal radiation therapy. External radiation therapy is generated when a machine delivers radiation to a specific part of the body with cancer. Internal occurs when radiation is placed within the tumor or cavities of the body. Side effects are common, because healthy cells are also damaged by radiation treatments.

Radiation can kill cancer cells, but it can also cause normal cells to develop into cancer. Secondary cancers can take up to twenty years to develop or as little as two to four years. Radiation to the chest area can create a restrictive cardiomyopathy that may lead to heart failure and can also induce breast cancer. Radiation to the head and neck frequently results in hypothyroidism. Whole-brain radiation can have a significant impact on cognition.

There are many natural ways to radiosensitize and increase the therapeutic effect of radiation. At least one week prior to radiation treatment, your child will benefit from entering a state of therapeutic ketosis. A patient should never undergo radiation treatment in a diabetic or prediabetic state. At the very minimum, feed your child no sugar and no grain. Studies show a huge difference between going through radiation with elevated blood sugar versus low blood sugar. I also recommend dosing shark liver oil for one week prior and during radiation treatment. Supplement dosing depends on the child's age and weight.

During Radiation (and Up to Three Weeks Following)[1]

- Ashwagandha, up to two capsules three times a day
- Berberine, up to 1,000 milligrams daily
- Vitamin E, up to 800 IU daily
- Vitamin A, up to 20,000 IU daily
- Turmeric, up to 2 grams daily
- Zinc citrate, 5 to 25 milligrams with each meal (reduces risk of mucositis)
- Fish oil
- Niacinamide, 500 to 1,000 milligrams up to three times a day (to increase tumor blood flow)
- Melatonin, up to 20 milligrams (protects the gastrointestinal mucosa and works as an antioxidant)
- High-dose IVC at the start of each week of radiation therapy

Chemotherapy

There are more than 100 different chemotherapy agents, and they are often combined with each other or with other cancer treatments like radiation or immunotherapy. Chemotherapy can be administered by mouth (orally), into a vein (intravenously), by injection into muscle, or by intrathecal injection into the spinal cord.

Chemotherapy has different treatment schedules. For example, treatment for ALL usually lasts at least two and a half years, while treatment for AML is shorter (about five months) but more intense. Treatment usually occurs in cycles. Some children may need more time to recover between cycles, but oncologists often want to avoid "chemo-delays," in order to prevent giving the cancer cells a "break" and opportunity to grow again.

While it's tempting to believe that chemotherapy kills cancer cells selectively, the truth is that very few chemotherapy drugs are selective. Some chemotherapy agents are much deadlier to healthy cells than to cancer cells.[2] The contribution of chemotherapy to the five-year survival rate for adults is estimated at a meager 2 percent.[3] (Those odds are better for children; leukemia is the most common childhood cancer, and it is mostly responsive to chemotherapy.) Chemotherapy is more effective with leukemias and lymphomas than it is with solid tumors. The same dose of chemotherapy may result in few noticeable side effects in one patient and lead to organ damage or death in another.

Integrative Support for Chemotherapy

The most important integrative support for chemotherapy, and cancer in general, is nutrition. At minimum, it is important that your child eliminates sugar and grain and eats a diet high in quality protein, healthy fat, and vegetables (Level 1 Nutrition). In many situations, I recommend that a child go through chemotherapy treatment in a therapeutic ketosis (Level 2 Nutrition). An exception would be treatment that lasts for years (such as the treatment for ALL); in that case it's best for a child to be in ketosis during IV chemotherapy days and eating a low-carbohydrate diet the rest of the time. For older children, I recommend fasting during IV chemotherapy days. Studies show that both fasting and a ketogenic diet during chemotherapy are safe and result in reduction of collateral effects of adjuvant chemotherapy and a better quality of life. Fasting or being in ketosis during chemotherapy helps protect healthy cells and decreases side effects.[4]

Try to have your older child fast for three days around their infusion, from day −1 to day 2. They should drink one to four quarts of fluid per day (half your child's body weight in pounds, in ounces of fluid) mostly in the form of broth, water, and tea, with an emphasis on hydration and electrolyte support. Coconut oil can be given to support ketogenic metabolism without compromising the fasting state. Between fasts, your child should eat a nutrient-dense, high-protein diet to aid in recovery.

In addition to fasting, I encourage patients who struggle to attain ketosis for their IV chemotherapy infusion to use exogenous ketones. (Not all exogenous ketones are created equal. Please see appendix D for recommendations.) In addition to nutrition, the following integrative therapies can work well alongside conventional treatment.

Mistletoe

Mistletoe injection therapy as an adjunct of chemotherapy has been shown to improve outcomes, improve tolerance, improve comfort, and decrease side effects, including fatigue.[5] In fact, mistletoe therapy is prescribed by more than 50 percent of doctors in Germany as an adjunct therapy. Although it is administered two to three times per week by subcutaneous injection, in my experience, most children, even as young as four years old, have no problem with the injections. You must work with a practitioner who has expertise in mistletoe therapy.

Low-Dose Naltrexone (LDN)

LDN is a potent immune therapy, synergistic with mistletoe. It can be formulated into a capsule or liquid or even a rapid-dissolve tablet. It is affordable and can sensitize cyclophosphamide, gemcitabine, and platinum chemotherapy drugs. LDN can interfere with narcotic pain medication, but it only has a half-life of six hours and therefore can be quickly stopped if narcotic pain meds are necessary. Ultra-low-dose options can be used even in patients who need to use narcotic pain medication.

L-glutamine

L-glutamine protects both the nerves and the mucous lining of the gastrointestinal tract. Chemotherapy-induced nerve and gut damage can be among the most painful side effects a child might experience, so it is worth doing whatever you can to ease this suffering. However, L-glutamine also warrants caution; I do not recommend administering the supplement daily, or at all, if your child has high lactate dehydrogenase lab results. It's thought L-glutamine may stimulate cancer cell growth under these conditions.

Fish Oil

Fish oil with omega-3 DHA is considered a chemosensitizer, meaning that it can help improve chemotherapy outcomes by regulating immune cell signaling and cytokines.

Mucositis Mouth Rinse

I use this mouth rinse for the prevention and treatment of mucositis. To make it, combine 5 grams L-glutamine powder, 1 cup water, and two to six crushed Gastrazyme pills from Biotics Research. Have your child sip, swish, and swallow all day. When lactate dehydrogenase is high, indicating infection, inflammation, or uncontrolled cancer, have your child swish and spit only, but not swallow. Again, it's thought that L-glutamine might stimulate cancer growth under these conditions, so this protocol is simply an abundance of caution.

Vitamin A

Vitamin A supports cell management and improves tumor response to chemotherapy and radiation. Use it short term in high doses (up to 100,000 IU) during intensive conventional treatment. Oncologists may get nervous about it causing liver toxicity and, while rare, that can happen. (Personally, I have never seen it happen, but I have seen liver toxicity caused by chemotherapy a lot.) You can ask your child's medical team to check vitamin A levels at any point.

Vitamin D3

Vitamin D3 plays an important role in preventing chemotherapy-induced intestinal mucositis. It also promotes cancer cell death and inhibits angiogenesis, the spread of cancer through making its own new blood vessels. Most kids (and most people) do not have sufficient levels of vitamin D. Vitamin D levels of at least 50 nanomoles per liter have been shown to reduce the risk of cancer, as well as help prevent relapse.[6] Many experts, including Dr. Paul Anderson, recommend levels of somewhere between 70 and 100 nanomoles per liter.[7] Dosing is dependent on age and weight and the level of nanomole per liter a child is starting at; I recommend 2,000 to 20,000 IU daily through treatment for most children. With high doses, in order to avoid hypercalcemia, vitamin D3 needs to be given with vitamin K2.

CBD/Full-Spectrum Hemp/Cannabis Oil

Depending on what location you live in and the legalities where you are, I recommend organic full-spectrum hemp oil, cannabis oil 1:1, or preferably both. These therapies are helpful for nausea, vomiting, pain, inflammation, anxiety, sleep, and graft-versus-host disease prevention and treatment. This is a powerful therapy to alleviate many common side effects through treatment instead of the frequently prescribed pharmaceutical alternatives.

High-dose IV Vitamin C
High-dose IVC both improves chemotherapy's efficacy and reduces side effects. Many oncologists will advise you that IVC reduces chemotherapy efficacy, even though there are multiple studies and decades of data demonstrating the opposite.[8] The prudent move (practically more than medically) in my opinion is to not administer high-dose IVC infusion within twenty hours either before or after chemotherapy treatments.

What to Avoid
Yes, there are integrative therapies and agents that must be avoided with certain chemotherapy drugs. It is imperative you work with a professional to clearly understand what these are and under what circumstances they should be avoided. It's important not to administer anything that uses the same liver detoxification pathways as the chemotherapy drugs. In general, the following are not recommended during treatment:

- Grapefruit, Valencia oranges
- St. John's wort
- High-sugar, high-carb diet
- High-dose selenium
- Quercetin (depending on type of chemotherapy)
- High-dose IVC on days of IV chemotherapy

Integrative Support for Specific Chemotherapies
How toxic is chemotherapy? It's toxic to nerve cells; vincristine is a common chemotherapy drug most known for this. It's toxic to heart cells, especially doxorubicin. It's toxic to rapidly growing cells like skin cells and the cells that line the GI tract. It's toxic to hair follicles. It's toxic to brain cells, causing the notorious "chemo brain." It's toxic to organs, such as the liver, kidneys, and lungs. It contributes to cancers, such as leukemia and lymphoma. It causes cancer cells to develop multidrug resistance. (Quercetin, turmeric, melatonin, and vitamin C can all help with this.)

Many families are instructed not to use integrative treatments when treating with chemotherapy for fear that the integrative treatments will get in the way of the chemotherapy's efficacy, especially in the case of high-dose antioxidants. However, studies continue to show that antioxidants are not a problem during chemotherapy.[9] That being said, it is very important to work closely with a metabolic oncology practitioner. Integrative support during chemotherapy can help make the chemotherapy agent more effective and less toxic. Less toxicity means fewer side effects during treatment and potentially fewer late effects in years to come. Late effects occur months to years after the chemotherapy treatment has been completed and may include heart damage, liver damage, and fertility issues.

Alkylating Agents

Alkylating agents interfere with the cancer's ability to reproduce itself by damaging DNA. They are commonly used for leukemia, lymphoma, sarcoma, and bone marrow transplant recipients. Side effects can include bone marrow toxicity, mucositis, secondary leukemias, nausea, vomiting, toxicity of organs, and hair loss.

Common alkylating agents include the following:

- Busulfan
- Thiotepa
- Melphalan
- Cyclophosphamide
- Temozolomide
- Cisplatin
- Oxaliplatin
- Carboplatin

Increase alkylating agents' effectiveness with the following:

- Quercetin
- Omega-3s
- Vitamin A
- Coenzyme Q10
- Low-dose naltrexone

Reduce alkylating agents' toxicity with the following:

- Omega-3s
- Ashwagandha
- Coenzyme Q10
- Melatonin (contraindicated in leukemia)
- Mushroom extract, such as the active hexose-correlated compound (AHCC) found in reishi and cordyceps

Exercise caution with turmeric, N-acetylcysteine, glutathione, dichloroacetate, and large doses of vitamin B6 or B12.

Magnesium, zinc, milk thistle, L-glutamine, vitamin A, and DCA can be helpful with carboplatin in particular.

Antimetabolites

Antimetabolites work by interfering with cancer cell replication and are most commonly used in leukemias. Side effects can include mucositis, elevated liver enzymes, joint pain, diarrhea, stomach pain, nausea, and vomiting. Avoid high doses of folic acid and glutathione during antimetabolite treatment since they can interfere with treatment efficacy.

Improve the effectiveness of antimetabolites with the following:

- Milk thistle
- L-glutamine
- Fish oil

Reduce the toxicity of antimetabolites with the following:

- Vitamin A
- Vitamin E
- Selenium

Antimetabolites and their integrative support include the following:

- 5-FU fluorourcil (5-FU); omega-3s; vitamins A, C, and E; L-glutamine. Avoid beta carotene and high-dose folic acid.
- Methotrexate. Avoid glutathione, high doses of folic acid, and oral vitamin C.
- Cytarabine. Prevent mouth sores with gastrazyme. Improve effectiveness with turmeric. Avoid vitamin B12.
- Gemcitabine. Support with quercetin and L-glutamine. Improve effectiveness with astragalus, quercetin, low-dose naltrexone, reishi, and B-complex vitamins. Avoid folate supplements.
- Mercaptopurine. Avoid quercetin and excess dairy.
- Fludarabine / cladribine / nelarabine.

Antitumor Antibiotics

Antitumor antibiotics work by interfering with DNA to prevent cancer cell division, and therefore replication. They are commonly used in treating pediatric leukemia, and side effects include nausea and vomiting, mucositis, bone marrow suppression, liver disease, skin rash, fever, joint pain, heart damage, painful urination, and digestive tract bleeding.

Antitumor antibiotics and their integrative support include the following:

- Daunorubicin
- Actinomycin-D
- Mitomycin
- Bleomycin. Can cause lung damage. Improve effectiveness with quercetin. Reduce toxicity with vitamins A, E, C, and selenium.
- Doxorubicin. Highly toxic to the heart muscles. Improve effectiveness with vitamins A and C, grape-seed extract OPCs, vitamin E, mistletoe, and quercetin. Reduce toxicity with melatonin, selenium, garlic, omega-3, milk thistle, vitamin E, and coenzyme Q10. Reduce toxicity to the heart specifically with grape-seed extract OPCs. Avoid N-acetyl-cysteine and glutathione.

Topoisomerase Inhibitors

Topoisomerase inhibitors work by preventing DNA and RNA from copying and replicating. They are commonly used in pediatric leukemias. Side effects include nausea and vomiting, diarrhea, stomach pain, weakness, fever, liver damage, hair loss, increased risk of secondary leukemias, and cardiac toxicity.

Topoisomerase inhibitors and their integrative support include the following:

- Etoposide. Improve effectiveness with vitamin A, quercetin, and melatonin. Avoid vitamin B12 and St. John's wort.
- Irinotecan. Can cause severe diarrhea. Treated with two to four capsules of charcoal up to twice daily (before and after the infusion) and slippery elm. Improve effectiveness with quercetin, melatonin, turmeric, milk thistle, selenium, and fish oil.
- Topotecan. Same integrative support as irinotecan.

Mitotic Inhibitors

Mitotic inhibitors are derived from natural substances, such as plants, and work by inhibiting cell division. They are commonly used in treating pediatric leukemia. Side effects include nerve damage and neuropathy, bone marrow suppression, nausea and vomiting, anemia, and hair loss.

Mitotic inhibitors and their integrative support include the following:

- Paclitaxel
- Vincristine

- Vinblastine. Can cause nerve toxicity. Prevent and treat with L-glutamine, vitamins B6 and B1, milk thistle, vitamin B12, acetyl-L-carnitine. Increase effectiveness with omega-3s, vitamins A, E, and C, and quercetin.

Tyrosine Kinase Inhibitors

Tyrosine kinase inhibitors work by blocking a family of enzymes known as tyrosine inhibitors. These drugs are more targeted than many chemotherapies to cancer cells specifically and are commonly used in treating pediatric leukemias. Side effects can include low white blood cell count, low platelets, nausea and vomiting, diarrhea, headache, muscle cramps, fluid retention, and depression.

Tyrosine kinase inhibitors and their integrative support include the following:

- Imatinib
- Sorafenib. Carries risk of bleeding. Improve efficacy and avoid toxicity with turmeric and melatonin. Avoid blood thinners.

Demethylating Agents

Demethylating agents work by destroying abnormally dividing cells in the bone marrow and are common in treating pediatric leukemias. Side effects include bleeding (from low platelets), body aches, chest pain, dizziness, feeling unusually cold, fever, hives, low appetite, mood changes, rash, stomach pain, breathing problem, weight loss, weakness, and irregular heart rate. Treatment with demethylating agents can be supported with mistletoe.

Demethylating agents include the following:

- Azacytidine
- Decitabine

L-asparaginase "PEG"

Asparaginase is an enzyme that breaks down the amino acid asparagine. Acute lymphocytic leukemia cells are unable to make their own asparagine, so asparaginase prevents the cancer cells from dividing and growing. Side effects of L-asparaginase include nausea and vomiting, poor appetite, stomach pain, weakness, allergic reaction, fatigue, diarrhea, mouth sores, pancreatitis, liver injury, and blood-clotting disorder. Supports include L-glutamine, gastrazyme, and cannabinoids.

Integrative Treatment for Radiation and Chemotherapy Side Effects

Having to sign papers that detail risks and side effects, including potential organ failure and death, is hard. I have had to do this too many times. But knowledge is power. Along with all these horrible risks and side effects are many ways to mitigate and reduce suffering. Try to stay focused on that. It will help you and help your child.

Below you will find integrative support for common side effects of chemotherapy and radiation. Some side effects are much more common to one or the other—for example, burns with radiation treatment or nausea and hair loss with chemotherapy—but many of the side effects and the treatments overlap.

As always, proceed with caution. Communicate fully and clearly with your child's oncology team and, if you have any doubt, wait. Nothing in this book is meant as a treatment guide. It is meant as a starting point for further investigation in collaboration with your integrated oncology practitioner and your child's oncology team.

Anemia

Anemia occurs when the bone marrow stops making enough red blood cells. This can happen as a result of chemotherapy or radiation and typically occurs a couple of days to a few weeks after treatment. Your child's oncology team may order a blood transfusion. They typically do this when hemoglobin reaches 7 grams per deciliter, but most kids will still have normal vital signs and no side effects with a hemoglobin of 7. It is best to transfuse when the patient is actually symptomatic (dizzy, weak), has abnormal vital signs, or hemoglobin drops below 7. Most kids need to be transfused even if they are asymptomatic with a hemoglobin of around 5.5 or 6. By assessing your child and lab work, you can avoid unnecessary transfusions and iron overload. Every transfusion your child undergoes will increase iron in their blood, and iron is very oxidizing and increases inflammation.

To help prevent or manage the effects of anemia, consider two capsules of shark liver oil one to three times daily, homemade bone broth, vitamin B12 injections or supplements, and marrow capsules from a quality supplement company.

Anosmia and Ageusia

Loss of smell (anosmia) and loss of taste (ageusia) are common after both chemotherapy and radiation, especially if the radiation was near the nasal and oral passage. Helpful therapies include vitamin B12 injections, N-acetyl-cysteine, acetyl-L-carnitine, and coenzyme Q10.

Appetite Loss

Loss of appetite is common during and after both chemotherapy and radiation. For this, I recommend herbal bitters, cannabis oil (where legal), and full-spectrum hemp oil in places where cannabis is not legal.

Burns

Radiation can cause severe burns to the skin and underlying tissue. Avoid any oil-based creams during radiation. Instead, use water-based calendula spray, aloe vera leaf gel, and topical colloidal silver. After radiation treatment is complete, I recommend calendula (again), vitamin A, and grape-seed extract oil creams.

Cognitive Impairment

Many parents notice that their kids have poor memory, poor concentration, and/or severe mood changes during chemotherapy. I remind parents to exercise as much patience and grace with their child as possible during treatment because, in addition to the extreme emotional toll that cancer takes, the brain is being heavily impacted by treatment. This is treatable, however, with detoxification and time. Tools for supporting chemo brain include omega-3 oils, B-complex vitamins, acetyl-L-carnitine, and full-spectrum hemp oil/CBD. With radiation therapy directly to the brain, cognitive impairment is a real concern. This we may not be able to prevent or treat.

Constipation

Constipation is another common side effect of both chemotherapy and radiation, especially for those in ketosis. Hydration is key. Magnesium (citrate) can help, as can enemas, aloe vera juice, vitamin C (to bowel tolerance), and castor oil packs over the lower abdomen. Consider supplements that combine natural stool softeners and laxatives such as Colon Motility Blend and LaxaBlend by Vitanica.

Dehydration

Dehydration is also common during treatment. Request intravenous rehydration with normal saline; often hospitals will use D5W, which is sugar water. Bone broth is also good for dehydration, as are sugar-free electrolyte drinks, such as the keto electrolyte powder packets from LMNT.

Dermatitis and Skin Rashes

Dermatitis and skin rashes are very common side effects of radiation and chemotherapy, especially during and following treatment. It often just takes time for these issues to resolve. You can help things along with topical calendula, topical and ingested turmeric, topical ozone cream, and aloe vera inner leaf gel.

Diarrhea

For diarrhea, try bone broth, electrolyte drinks (without sugar or artificial colors), probiotics, and intravenous rehydration with normal saline. Charcoal can also be helpful, but do not use it in conjunction with other supplements and medications. (Charcoal soaks up what it comes in contact with, preventing the body from absorbing other supplements and medications.)

Dry Mouth

It is common for patients to experience dry mouth after undergoing radiation to the neck or jaw. Artificial saliva products, such as sprays and lozenges can be helpful. Just be sure that they don't contain sugar and artificial flavors.

Fatigue

Fatigue is probably one of the most common side effects for both chemotherapy and radiation. If it's appropriate for your child's situation, mistletoe can greatly help with fatigue. You can also use 500 to 1,000 milligrams of L-carnitine one to three times per day, omega-3 fatty acids, B vitamins, ashwagandha, and an intravenous drip of Myers' cocktail IV or Poly MVA (either IV or oral). Chinese ginseng can work well for older kids (I avoid ginseng with younger kids as it can be too stimulating). Finally, although it can be difficult for patients to muster the energy, even small amounts of movement and exercise can aid greatly in reducing fatigue.

Hair Loss

Hair loss is usually unavoidable with certain chemotherapies and with radiation to the skull. Oral or topical vitamin E, topical vitamin C, and topical organic castor oil combined with scalp stimulation with a baby bristle brush can help. Consider cool cap therapy to help prevent loss, though not for every type of cancer, and not for radiation, only chemotherapy. Cool cap therapy or scalp cooling systems work by narrowing the blood vessels beneath the skin of the scalp. This reduces the amount of chemotherapy that reaches those hair follicles and may help prevent hair loss. Cool cap therapy is not advised for systemic cancers like leukemia and lymphoma. However, those with a solid tumor should ask their oncology team about it. Few hospitals will offer it to patients, and most pediatric hospitals do not. You can do a DIY version of this by buying cool caps yourself.

Headache

Headaches can occur during treatment. Before reaching directly for acetaminophen or ibuprofen, I recommend trying vitamin B2 (riboflavin), magnesium, hydration with electrolytes, or full-spectrum hemp oil.

Heartburn

Disturbance to the gut from chemotherapy can cause heartburn. I do not recommend proton-pump inhibitors for long-term use. Instead, try deglycyrrhizinated licorice chewable tablets and digestive enzymes or bitters.

Insomnia

I can't emphasize enough how important it is to protect your child's sleeping schedule through treatment. To help, I recommend eliminating blue light exposure before bed and adding melatonin (though not if your child is being treated for leukemia), chamomile tea, and full-spectrum hemp oil, or CBD or cannabis oil if it is legal where you are.

Heart Damage

Certain chemotherapy drugs are known to cause cardiac toxicity both during treatment and as a late effect. To best protect the heart, I recommend omega-3 fatty acids, grape-seed extract OPCs, up to 300 milligrams daily of coenzyme Q10, up to 400 IU daily of vitamin E, and L-carnitine.

Kidney Damage

Many chemotherapies and supporting medications, such as antiviral drugs, are hard on the kidneys. You can protect and repair your child's kidneys by always keeping them hydrated. Supplement daily with up to 300 milligrams coenzyme Q10; R-alpha-lipoic acid; up to 1 gram N-acetylcysteine; up to 2,000 milligrams, daily quercetin; ½ teaspoon baking soda, and celery, cilantro, and parsley juice.

Leukopenia

Leukopenia, a lower-than-normal white blood cell count, can be a side effect of both chemotherapy and radiation. With chemotherapy, white blood cell counts tend to fall approximately eleven to thirteen days after IV chemotherapy. It is imperative to be mindful that your child is prone to infections during that time and may get something called neutropenic fever. A drug called Neupogen (or Neulasta) is sometimes used to stimulate the bone marrow to recover faster. Be very cautious of this drug and discuss with your team if it is necessary; it has many immediate and long-term side effects, including leukemia. If your child must take Neupogen/Neulasta, Claritin can significantly help alleviate bone pain.

For leukopenia, try shark liver oil two to three times per day, astragalus, vitamin A (up to 50,000 IU daily), fermented wheat germ extract, and mistletoe for those for whom it is indicated. You can also cycle doses of germanium sesquioxide, 100 to 200 milligrams with food for two days on and five days off.

Lung Injury or Pneumonitis

Lung injury is common if radiation is directed near the lung fields. It usually begins between one and six months after treatment and can cause shortness of breath and chest pain. Certain chemotherapy drugs also have a potential for lung toxicity. Consider nebulized *Helleborus* (D12 or D6), turmeric, R-alpha-lipoic acid, and grape-seed extract. You can also treat with nebulized glutathione and high-dose N-acetylcysteine, up to 3 to 9 grams per day.

Mucositis

Mucositis is inflammation of the mucosa resulting in sores from the mouth all the way down the throat, esophagus, stomach, and rectum.

You can both prevent and treat these. I like to mix 1 cup of deuterium-depleted water and 5 grams of L-glutamine with two to six crushed tablets of Gastrazyme and have the patient swish and swallow all day to both prevent and heal mucositis. Other prevention and treatment options include the following:

- Vitamin U, such as Gastrazyme by Biotics Research, two to six tablets daily[10]
- Vitamin E, 200 to 800 IU
- L-glutamine, up to 10 grams per day but typically for a child 3 to 5 grams per day
- Deglycyrrhizinated licorice extract
- Magic mouthwash (by prescription, for pain)
- Coconut oil or coconut oil mixed with CBD oil

Nausea

Nausea is probably one of the most common side effects of both chemotherapy and radiation. Your child's oncologist will have a list of antinausea medications to try; you can also try the following natural remedies:

- Ginger, in the form of liquid (for little ones), ginger chews, or capsules
- Cannabis works very well, if you are in a location where it is legal
- Full-spectrum hemp oil, such as those from Twisted River Farms, with legal amounts of THC where legal
- Homeopathic nux vomica

Nerve Injury

Nerve damage, also known as neuropathy, is a potential side effect that can arise from both chemotherapy and radiation treatments. Nerve injury can cause various symptoms, such as tingling, numbness, pain, and weakness in the affected areas. Neuropathy can often be prevented or reversed. The following can help:

- Vitamin B12
- Vitamin B1
- Acetyl-L-carnitine, 1 to 3 grams up to three times daily
- Vitamin B6
- N-acetylcysteine

- L-glutamine
- Omega-3s
- Poly MVA by mouth
- IV formulations with key nutrients, especially Poly MVA
- Wet sock treatment: mix a 1:1 dilution of vinegar and put it on warm feet and cover with dry wool socks and go to bed

Organ Damage

Organ damage from chemotherapy or radiation is unfortunately common and ranges from mild to severe. The following therapies can help prevent heart, lung, kidney, and liver damage.

- Ashwagandha
- Coenzyme Q10 in high doses
- Melatonin 10 to 20 milligrams
- *Boswellia* in high doses
- MCT oil
- Omega-3s for brain injury
- Being in therapeutic ketosis or fasting during radiation

Platelet Damage

Both radiation and chemotherapy can affect your child's platelet count. If your child's platelets fall below 20, your doctor will order a transfusion to reduce the risk of severe bleeding. It's valuable to reduce the need for transfusions. The following supplements are helpful:

- Papaya leaf extract
- Shark liver oil
- Sesame oil (you can sneak this into food)
- High-dose IV vitamin C

Weight Loss

Cachexia is characterized by a severe and involuntary loss of weight, muscle mass, and appetite, which can lead to weakness and fatigue. This condition can have a significant impact on a patient's overall well-being. Early detection and intervention are crucial to managing cachexia and supporting the patient's nutritional needs throughout their treatment journey. Your team will likely recommend your child consume "nutrition" shakes, like Pedia-Sure. The following is a healthier way to manage weight loss:

- ½ teaspoon to 1 tablespoon of MCT oil every hour
- Increase EPA oils (fish oils)
- Anti-Cachexia Formula (see appendix B)
- Anti-Cachexia Smoothie (see appendix B)

Post-Treatment Healing

Ending conventional oncology treatment can be extraordinarily confusing. For many families, this is a time of immense relief and gratitude because your child is considered in remission. For other families, however, the end of treatment might not mean that at all. Many pediatric cancer patients never attain remission. So the end of treatment might mean that your child has a stable disease and needs to continue certain medications indefinitely. This is the reality of pediatric cancer.

Regardless of your child's situation, the end of treatment can be a complicated time. You might find yourself scrambling for a new normal. From my experience, I find that the first six months following the end of conventional treatment are actually the hardest. Now that you have some time to breathe, fears of relapse may surface and start to settle in your mind. You and your family members may be wondering what life will be like now. And people you know might be celebrating—and expecting you to celebrate—that "it's over." You might experience intense, confusing, and very uncomfortable feelings. You might wonder why you feel so sad when you are "supposed" to feel blessed and happy that treatment is over. You may slowly come to realize that nothing is ever quite over. It might never feel easy. You, your child, and the rest of your family are moving into a new phase of existence.

Many families are advised that monthly blood work or imaging is all that is necessary at this point. This is where conventional oncology truly fails. Post–conventional oncology care should involve so much more—it should be comprehensive. You deserve to know how to support your child and not only monitor for relapse, but truly help them heal. In the next chapter, I'll address the broken terrain that led to a cancer diagnosis, as well as focus on detoxification and healing the gut.

I think one reason my daughter was able to withstand more treatment and a second bone marrow transplant (many can't) is because we were extremely dedicated to healing her gut and detoxifying her body each time she completed treatment. It is hard to think about—what if my child relapses?—but I'm sorry to say, it's an important question. And it's one reason why it's so essential to take the business of healing your child's whole body so seriously.

Individualized detoxification and healing the gut are going to be a part of your new normal. Upon a child's initial cancer diagnosis, the focus is identifying the best treatment, support of that treatment, and stability of disease or remission. That does not mean detoxification and gut healing have no role in that phase, but they take a back seat. Once the disease is stable, or your child has no evidence of disease, it's time to put more energy into detoxification and healing the gut—and healing the broken terrain that led to the development of cancer in the first place.

CHAPTER 10

Detoxify

What does the word *detoxification* even mean? It seems like everywhere I turn, I see advertisers claiming that their products support "detoxification." It's a seductive marketing strategy—after all, who *doesn't* want to detoxify? If only it were as easy as taking a pill and waiting for toxins to pour out of your body so you could once again operate at full capacity.

In my opinion, detoxification is both simpler and more complex than purchasing natural health products and waiting for the miracle to happen. Detoxification isn't something you *do* to your body. Detoxification is something *your body* does all the time—all day long, every day, even while we sleep. That's the real miracle: Our bodies have evolved over millions of years to deal with all sorts of waste products in many different ways: respiration, metabolism, urination, defecation, via the kidneys, the liver, the intestines, the lymphatic system, the skin, and so much more. When you think about it this way, it seems odd that we think we might improve upon this with a coconut-water-and-spinach detox smoothie.

Detoxification is happening all the time. But assaults on our bodies are also happening all the time, so it's a good idea to support this miraculous process to the greatest extent possible. The best exogenous detoxification methods will support and improve upon the ongoing endogenous detoxification that our bodies engage in every second of every day. Even if your child is sick with cancer and their detoxification pathways are compromised, their body is still working incredibly hard and doing incredibly well to carry out its basic functions. It's important to acknowledge this: Even if your child is very ill, there is still more going right than going wrong.

Detoxification is such a critical part of healing for the pediatric cancer patient. Toxic substances can be a major contributing factor to cancer in the first place. Many cancers are caused by substances found in the environment.[1] Some children are more vulnerable than others. For example, children with the PON1 mutation are more vulnerable to carcinogenic pesticide and herbicide exposure.[2]

In addition to substances that may have contributed to the development of cancer, it's important to understand that conventional cancer treatments, including chemotherapy, radiation, and most immunotherapies, are also extremely toxic. It is important to support the body in effectively moving those toxins out. It is also essential that detoxification strategies become part of your child's lifestyle in order to reduce the risk of relapse or late effects. The main detoxification organs that I cover in this chapter are the liver and the kidneys as well as the lymphatic system, skin, lungs, and digestive tract.

Liver Support

The liver is a master detoxifier. It works as a filter, separating out metabolic by-products and breaking them down so they can then be further filtered by the kidneys. The liver helps process hormones, chemicals, and heavy metals. It works in two stages. The first transforms enzymes into free radicals. Then the antioxidant glutathione attaches to the free radicals and neutralizes them.

The liver bears the greatest burden of processing chemotherapy agents. You might notice your child's liver enzymes are elevated during chemotherapy treatment. The liver is also where many children with cancer have suboptimal pathways to begin with. (This situation can be identified through epigenetic testing; see chapter 3 and appendix A.) Compromised liver detoxification allows chemicals like glyphosate to build up in the body. Then, with the addition of chemotherapy, the liver may experience further buildup.

Conventional lab tests can help you identify if your child's liver is becoming irritated from cancer treatment. The labs you should look at are AST, ALT, GGT, Alk Phos, INR, PT, and bilirubin (see chapter 3 and appendix A). Abnormality in these results will often mean that the liver is overloaded and irritated. General liver detoxification support can include the use of castor oil packs, milk thistle, N-acetylcysteine, glutathione, dandelion root, and methylation supplements.

Castor Oil Packs

Castor oil can help support the liver when its detoxification pathways become overburdened. I used castor oil packs three times a week while my daughter was undergoing treatment known to irritate the liver, and daily when I had evidence through lab tests that her liver was irritated.

To make a castor oil pack, you will need a piece of flannel cloth, a vinyl hot water bottle, warm water for the bottle, organic castor oil, and two towels or pillowcases. Ideally, the linens should be organic and free of scents and dyes; something that has been through the wash many times is preferable to buying something new that has been recently treated with chemicals. The castor oil should be cold-pressed and free of pesticides and chemicals. Some drugstore brands will be rinsed with hexane for extraction. Your best bet is to buy organic castor oil in a glass bottle.

Position your child on their left side, so their liver (on the right side) will be fully exposed to the castor oil treatment. Place the towel or pillowcase on the treatment area. Next, saturate the piece of flannel with castor oil, so it is wet but not dripping, and position it on the skin above the liver. (Be forewarned that castor oil is very sticky.) Cover the flannel castor oil pack with a vinyl hot water bottle, being careful not to burn your child's skin by overheating the water. The warm water will help the castor oil penetrate the skin. Next, wrap another towel or pillowcase around your child's body, covering the flannel and the hot water bottle and holding everything in place. You can also stack pillows on your child's right side to hold the pack in a comfortable position.

I like to keep castor oil packs in place for an hour, but even twenty minutes can be worthwhile. After the treatment, your child's skin can be cleaned with a solution of baking soda dissolved in water, about two teaspoons per quart of warm water. Save all your materials for future use, but be aware that the oil will eventually become rancid and you will need to replace anything that has come in contact with it.

Milk Thistle and Dandelion Root

The plant milk thistle is commonly used for liver detoxification support. Its seeds contain a flavonoid called silymarin that can be extracted by grinding the seeds. Silymarin has powerful antioxidant and anti-inflammatory properties, helping to regenerate and maintain high levels of glutathione in the liver. Glutathione helps the liver detox.

Dandelion root also enhances the liver's detoxification capacity. The polysaccharides in the dandelion are known to reduce stress on the liver and help filter harmful compounds. Dandelion root can also be very supportive of the kidneys.

Glutathione, N-acetylcysteine, and Methylation Nutrients

Glutathione is the mother of all antioxidants and a master detoxifier. It is a simple combination of three amino acids—cysteine, glycine, and glutamine—and the body produces it naturally all the time. Many pediatric cancer patients have impaired epigenetics that can lead to suboptimal glutathione production, which can contribute to the development of cancer to begin with, as well as impaired capacity of the liver to detoxify from conventional treatment.[3] Chronic liver inflammation, which your child might experience through treatment, depletes their body of glutathione.[4]

Studies show that glutathione reduces oxidative stress-induced liver damage.[5] Basically, the more you can support the body in synthesizing glutathione, the better the liver's ability to detox. That said, glutathione is not well absorbed as a supplement; IV, inhaled, or oral liposomal glutathione are good options. Since glutathione tastes like rotten eggs, nebulized glutathione can be a better bet for kids.

On a related note, N-acetylcysteine (NAC) is a small protein that can aid in restoring intracellular glutathione. NAC has been shown to reduce liver toxicity and bilirubin during stem cell transplant. (Lower bilirubin is associated with improved survival.[6]) An NAC supplement is something you might consider, especially if your child will be undergoing a stem cell transplant. Methylation nutrients, including methylated folate, vitamin B6, and vitamin B12, are also critical in the production of glutathione.

I like to apply glutathione liver support as a "pulse therapy." That means I choose one glutathione-related supplement and use it for a month. Then I might stop the supplement and use only castor oil packs for a month. Then I might consider adding a supplement back in. Please note, however, that children should *not* take NAC or glutathione long term, because doing so can result in low zinc levels and has even been linked to liver cancer. This type of supplementation needs to be done under the guidance of an experienced clinician.

Gallbladder Support

The liver makes bile and the gallbladder stores it. The gallbladder then releases bile into the small intestine to break down fat. Bile salts bind to fat-soluble toxins and carry them out of the body through the stool. This is a major mechanism of moving fat-soluble toxins out of the body, so a healthy functioning gallbladder is extremely important.

Because the gallbladder and liver work closely together, they are supported by similar nutrition, supplements, and detoxification methods. (The lab work you might look at will be bilirubin, alkaline phosphatase, alanine transaminase, and aspartate transaminase.) The only additional support to add for the gallbladder is digestive enzymes, which help the gallbladder in breaking down fat. This can be part of a gut-healing protocol, which is essential for patients who have been through any type of conventional cancer treatment. When following a low-carbohydrate, high-quality-fat diet, as I recommend, digestive enzymes are key to help the body break down that fat.

Kidney Support

The kidneys filter waste, including medication by-products, for excretion. Kidneys also help the body regulate fluid and electrolyte balance and release three important hormones: erythropoietin, which stimulates the bone marrow to make red blood cells; renin, which regulates blood pressure; and calcitriol, the active form of vitamin D3, which helps maintain calcium for bones and for regulating parathyroid levels. Children undergoing cancer treatment will have their kidney function tested often because the kidneys can so easily be harmed. The labs you should keep an eye on are creatinine, blood urea nitrogen (BUN), and urinalysis.

Dandelion and marshmallow root can help support kidney function and detoxification. Human studies suggest that dandelion has diuretic activity, meaning it can increase the kidneys' ability to filter toxins. Dandelion root tea is an easy way to gently support kidney filtration; dandelion root can also be taken as an extract. Marshmallow also supports kidney function through its diuretic effects. It eases inflammation in the urinary tract, supporting both the kidneys and the bladder. Many gut-repair supplements include marshmallow root, and it is easily taken as a tea or extract.

Digestive Support

The key to digestive tract detoxification is daily healthy bowel movements because the intestinal tract plays a major role in detoxification. In order to have a daily bowel movement, however, you need proper gut health. An unhealthy gut can both contribute to cancer and be the result of cancer treatment.[7] Typical cancer drugs, including antibiotics, steroids, and chemotherapy agents, completely ruin gut health, and it can take years to restore it. (In general, use of antibiotics under the age of two or multiple courses of antibiotics under the age of ten correlate with poor health outcomes.[8]) The labs you should keep an eye on are GI-Map, OATs test, and stool testing.

Regular bowel movements also require proper hydration. Even mild dehydration can cause constipation, especially in infants and children.[9] A general rule of thumb is to drink half your body weight (in pounds) in ounces of water every day. Water quality is important; I recommend using a good filtration system.

Magnesium is also important in the regulation of bowel movements. Magnesium draws water into the intestines, working as an osmotic laxative, which stimulates bowel motility. Magnesium is considered a safe and effective treatment for constipation in children.[10] Magnesium citrate is best for constipation but should be used carefully. Magnesium glycinate is better for stress relief, anxiety, and muscle relaxation. Combining the two gives a gentle laxative effect—more than just using citrate alone.

Dry cupping and abdominal wall massage can be as effective in children as standard laxative therapy. Dry cupping is a manual therapy that involves positioning a cup on the skin and creating a vacuum to apply negative pressure. The negative pressure increases blood flow to the area. You can purchase cupping sets or go to a practitioner.

Binders, which can be taken orally as a pill or powder, can also be an important part of intestinal detoxification. Binders are so called because they bind toxins and remove them via the digestive tract so that they are not reabsorbed into the body. They can be specific to certain toxins or heavy metals and can help reduce stress on detoxification organs, such as the liver and kidneys, as well as help prevent an inflammatory reaction or Herxheimer reaction. (A Herxheimer reaction is a natural process triggered by the prevalence of endotoxins when harmful microorganisms or bacteria die off en masse.)

For example, charcoal is a simple binder. It is broad spectrum but is effective in soaking up many toxins. Bentonite clay is another effective binder. GI Detox, manufactured by the company Biocidin, combines charcoal, zeolite clay, and aloe. Humic and fulvic acids can be effective for detoxing glyphosate.[11] Binders can also slow down the digestive tract, so you need to be careful with dosing when constipation is already present.

Lymphatic Support

The lymphatic system is a major part of the body's detoxification system and includes the spleen, thymus, adenoids, and tonsils, connected by capillaries, vessels, and hundreds of lymph nodes. Its main role is to transport lymphocytes and help fight infections and protect against toxins. Your child's CBC lab test will show if they have healthy ranges of lymphocytes and a healthy ratio (2:1) of neutrophils to lymphocytes.

Rebounding—aka jumping on a trampoline—is an excellent way for kids to reduce lymphatic congestion. If you can, buy your child a large outdoor trampoline. Most kids will start jumping and playing on it without any prompting on your part. The gravitational pull from bouncing results in lymphatic drainage in just a few minutes. In winter, a small indoor rebounder is also an option, but not as fun.

Lymphatic massage or manual lymphatic drainage has been used for years to help with lymphatic drainage. Specialized lymphatic massage therapists learn techniques to help with their hands support lymphatic drainage. This is especially useful in conditions with edema or inflammation. Lymphedema occurs when lymph nodes need to be removed or have been damaged from cancer treatment. This can create a sluggish lymphatic drainage and regular lymphatic massage can help support the movement of the fluid that accumulates.

Dry brushing also promotes lymphatic drainage, although I find that it can be challenging with younger children. With a dry brush (an inexpensive natural bristle brush will do), gently brush their skin in a circular motion toward the heart for a few minutes before they take a shower or bath. Lymphatic massage can also help reduce swelling.[12]

Respiratory Support

Starting with the nose and ending in the lungs, the respiratory system forms its own protective barrier to help keep particles out of the lungs. Making sure your child's nasal passage is clear and teaching your child proper slow, deep breathing is essential to respiratory detoxification. There are no labs, per se, but keep an eye on oxygen saturation, heart rate, and lung auscultation (listening with a stethoscope).

Let's pause for a moment on the importance of breathing. Most of us don't give our breathing much thought, but it can play a vital role in calming our nervous systems, managing pain, and detoxifying our lungs.[13] The same is true for our children. Deep breathing, or "breathwork," involves taking slower and deeper breaths, which can be extremely valuable for a child with cancer. Cancer treatments can often cause pain, feelings of nervousness, and many other strong emotions. Breathwork offers a powerful tool to cope with these challenges. Deep breathing exercises can help children relax and reduce anxiety, providing a sense of calm during medical procedures and treatments. Moreover, breathwork empowers children to regain a sense of control over their bodies and emotions, promoting a positive and proactive approach to their healing process. Intentional breathwork methods also support healthy lung function and overall well-being.

The Owaken app or a HeartMath device can be connected to a phone, offering personalized guidance. The Buteyko method is specifically designed to help people transition from mouth breathing to nasal breathing. Mouth breathing has been linked to facial deformities, growth issues (which some children may experience post-treatment), gum disease, and crooked teeth. Through simple breathing exercises practiced every day for four to six weeks, the Buteyko method can restore natural breathing patterns and promote healthy nasal breathing habits. It is also excellent for the lungs.

Cupping and chest compression can help remove the buildup of excess heat in the lungs and clear the lungs of congestion, phlegm, and fluids. You can buy a cupping set that is easy to use at home and safe for children. (Avoid cupping if your child's platelets are low from disease or treatment.) Cupping is excellent therapy if your child has a cold or cough that could lead to infection in the lungs.

Helleborus is a perennial herb sometimes referred to as Christmas rose. It is often used as an adjunct cancer therapy (see chapter 7), and is also excellent for lung therapy when inhaled. Ask your integrative clinician for a prescription and dosage for your child. Jade Windscreen is a Chinese herbal formula composed of three herbs—astragalus root, atractylodes rhizome, and siler root—that helps support the immune system and works particularly well if your child has a cold that affects the lungs. Mix it with a little water (it's slightly sweet) and offer it to your child every other day for four to eight weeks.

Skin Support

Our skin is our largest organ and the body's defense system. It creates a barrier against the outside world, protecting us from toxins, viruses, bacteria, and other substances that can harm us. We detoxify through our skin by sweating; all the ways to promote detoxification through the skin include sweating. This one is simple: exercise. Kids love to play hard—let them.

Infrared sauna affects all the detoxification organs. At the most basic level, saunas create heat to help us sweat. This is excellent for skin detoxification. Infrared sauna also penetrates deeper than the skin, however, because infrared light is perceived by the body as heat, making your child's body sweat at lower temperatures, and is therefore better tolerated. (Always check with your health practitioner before considering a sauna for kids with shunts or ports or feeding tubes.) Build your child up slowly with low heat for short amounts of time, gradually increasing so that they sweat for at least ten minutes. Choose a sauna with low EMFs.

Baths and foot soaks are a soothing detox method and, if warm enough, will cause sweating. Adding Epsom salts will promote relaxation and magnesium absorption. Baths and foot soaks are not nearly as effective as infrared sauna, but they can be a positive and relaxing routine for your child, especially at bedtime.

Detoxing Specific Substances

The first step in supporting detoxification from a specific substance is to remove the exposure. Once we have removed the exposure, or controlled it as much as possible, then it makes sense to focus on the best detoxification methods for the given exposure. I say this with a huge caveat, which is one of the most infuriating and frustrating aspects of childhood cancer: There are so *many* toxic substances in our world—and those who profit from them are rarely held accountable for the harm they cause—that it can be difficult to determine a causal relationship between exposure to a given carcinogen and the development of cancer. On the other hand, in the case of some carcinogens (for example, cigarettes and, increasingly, glyphosate), there is a clear epidemiological and biological science drawing a causal link to cancer, and there are increasingly targeted tests and other methods to establish strong correlations that will help you target your efforts to support your child's health and healing.[14]

Glyphosate (aka Roundup)

One of the most important things you can do for your entire family's overall health is switch your diet to organic and non-GMO foods. Do not use Roundup on your lawn, and politely ask your neighbors to do the same.

Switch out your toiletries to nontoxic products. Glyphosate is water-soluble and therefore relatively easy to eliminate out of the body.

The two most effective ways I have found to detoxify glyphosate are through the use of infrared sauna (every other day) and Cellcore's HM-ET Binder, which contains humic and fulvic acid (as well as zeolite, and broccoli sprouts), to bind glyphosate in the GI tract and accelerate its excretion.[15] I also recommend a daily shot of organic sauerkraut juice for glyphosate detox.[16]

Mold

Mold can cause an acute or chronic inflammatory response with multiple symptoms. Immunocompromised patients are at a higher risk from mold exposure and fungal infections.[17] Your child's oncologist may prescribe an antifungal medication to be used prophylactically during treatment if your child is immunocompromised.

With mold, it's important to identify the source, which isn't always easy. It can also be difficult to mitigate mold without spreading it further. Reach out to your state public health department for information and a list of contractors.

You can help your child detox from mold with a gentle daily binder like GI Detox, but be sure not to give it to them with food or other supplements, because a binder will bind other things as well, including medication and nutrients. The rest of the process can get complicated, in part because myco-toxins can launch an inflammatory response or infection elsewhere in the body. I highly recommend working with an integrative practitioner who has specific experience with mold exposure, children, and cancer.

Chemotherapy

Many conventional oncologists will tell you that chemotherapy will stay in your child's body for only a matter of days, or even hours. But this assumes that all your child's detoxification pathways and organs are functioning opti-mally, which is rarely the case if your child has cancer.

Detox from chemotherapy might involve infrared sauna, rebounding, binders, and hydration, but you need to be careful about timing during treat-ment. Do not administer binders or sauna less than forty-eight hours before or after chemotherapy injections. If your child takes oral chemotherapy daily for months to years, speak to your integrative practitioner about timing of detox modalities. Once conventional treatment is completely done, you can focus more on detoxification from chemotherapy.

EMF Exposure

It is said that cell phones are the cigarettes of the twenty-first century, and this means all our kids are smoking. The year 2019 brought a whole new toxic assault into your child's world: 5G. Many studies have found harmful biologic or health effects from exposure to 5G.[18] Many scientists believe we have enough evidence to consider it a known human carcinogen, and the relationship between brain cancer and EMF exposure is especially high.[19] After several elementary age kids in California were diagnosed with cancer within months of each other, Sprint shut down a cell phone tower.[20]

Are you starting to feel overwhelmed? I know, this one gets me, too, because 5G is everywhere. Avoiding it is becoming nearly impossible. What can you do to reduce your child's exposure? The biggest exposures in your home are from Wi-Fi, cell phones, and smart meters. Here are some thoughts:

- Limit exposure by setting rules about iPhone, iPad, and computer use.
- Use EMF-reducing covers; these are not perfect but they're better than nothing.
- Hardwire all of your internet connections. If this isn't an option, turn your router off at night.
- Keep your smart phone on airplane mode and turn your data off when you are not using it or expecting a phone call. (You can do this at night; your alarm will still work. Better yet, keep your phone out of your bedroom at night and get a regular alarm.)
- Avoid streaming on your phone.
- Avoid a smart meter if you can. If you cannot opt out of the smart meter, then use a smart meter shield.
- Be aware of the other devices in your home. Check the EMFs of your printers, blenders, and other "smart" appliances. Keep these turned off when you are not using them.
- Have an electrician install a kill switch so you can avoid EMFs in your child's bedroom at night or turn the breaker to their room off every night.
- Invest in an EMF meter to measure the EMFs inside your house and around devices.

- Invest in an EMF-reducing device for your home or your child's room.
- Do not use AirPods or Bluetooth.
- Use high-quality blue-light-blocking glasses when using your devices.

Foods That Support Detoxification

Certain foods are known for their detoxification properties. It's easy to sneak most of these foods into smoothies, and if your child has an NG or G tube, it's even easier to sneak them into their diet. That said, it's also important to expose your children to these foods so they can develop a taste for them as they grow up.

Beets and Beet Greens

Beets contain betaine and betalain, which help the liver process fat. They also contain folate, which is important for the methylation pathway, and the greens contain vitamins C and A, which are both beneficial to the immune system. Beets are high in carbohydrates, so a small amount goes a long way. Beets are good roasted, and beet greens can be added to smoothies.

Beets can also be fermented, taking this wonderful detox food a step further by introducing gut-healing probiotics. My mom makes fermented beet juice (kvass), and my daughter drinks it every other day. Be aware that many online recipes for beet kvass include unnecessary ingredients and overcomplicate the process. All you need is beets, salt, and water.

Dandelion

Dandelions are edible! Often when we think of dandelions, we think of getting rid of them, but they are an amazing detox food. You can use the dandelion greens out of your yard if it has not been sprayed with pesticides for several years. Both the greens and the roots can be added to salads or smoothies or steeped into a tea. Dandelions support liver detoxification and digestive tract stimulation.

Lemons

You may have heard that warm water with a squeeze of lemon is a great way to start the day. I agree! Starting your day with lemon stimulates your liver and gallbladder and every part of the lemon aids in detoxification. The zest of a lemon contains a terpene, which gives us that beautiful smell, that has anticancer and chemoprotective activity.[21] Lemon juice is also high in vitamin C, which aids in the detoxification of heavy metals.

If your child consumes too much THC from hemp or cannabis oil, you can decrease the psychoactive side effects by giving them a lemon tea. Cut the lemon in half, squeeze it, shave some zest, and then pour hot water over it.

Cruciferous Vegetables

Cruciferous vegetables include broccoli and broccoli sprouts, cauliflower, cabbage, arugula, Brussels sprouts, and bok choy. These brassica family vegetables contain an active compound called sulforaphane, one of the most potent antioxidants and detoxifiers. In multiple studies it has been shown to support glutathione synthesis, improve mitochondrial functions, and reduce inflammation.[22] Sulforaphane has also been shown to be chemoprotective and possibly help with apoptosis. Some sulforaphane-rich foods include the following:

- Arugula
- Bok choy
- Broccoli
- Broccoli sprouts
- Brussels sprouts
- Cabbage
- Cauliflower
- Daikon radish
- Kale
- Kohlrabi
- Radishes
- Turnips
- Watercress

Broccoli sprouts have the most benefit and are easily blended if you're using a feeding tube.

Animal Proteins

Animal proteins contain amino acids that are essential for our detoxification pathways. These foods include eggs, wild salmon, organ meats, stocks and bone broths, and high-quality whey protein. Eggs are incredibly easy to incorporate into your child's diet for any meal of the day. Whey protein is also easy to sneak into a smoothie or cup of bone broth. Quality sourcing is essential. Only feed your child organic, non-GMO, and preferably grass-fed and grass-finished protein. Eggs should be from free-range, pasture-raised chickens. Seafood should be wild-caught.

Chlorella and Chlorophyll

Chlorella is a green algae that is often available as a powder, which is easy to incorporate into a smoothie. Chlorella is chemoprotective, and studies have shown it to induce cancer cell death in the liver.[23] It is also a natural heavy metal detoxifier, detoxifying as well as inhibiting the absorption of heavy metals such as arsenic, mercury, and lead.

Chlorophyll is the green pigment found in plants and algae. In several studies, it has been shown to inhibit cancer progression by targeting pathways involved in cancer cell cycle progression, invasion, and angiogenesis.[24] The quality of any chlorella and chlorophyll you purchase is extremely important.

Unfortunately, we live in a toxic world, and we are all exposed to higher-than-ideal levels of toxicity throughout our lives. As for our kids, their toxic burden likely contributed in at least some way to the development of their cancer. Considering that cancer treatment itself can be highly toxic, it is that much more important to support the body's detoxification after undergoing conventional treatment. The best approach to supporting a child's detoxification, beyond foundational measures such as hydration and sweating, is by working with an integrative oncology specialist who can help interpret your child's epigenetic hiccups and recommend individualized practices to help their body detoxify more effectively.

CHAPTER 11

Restore the Gut

CHEMOTHERAPY, RADIATION, STEROIDS, AND ANTIBIOTICS ADVERSELY affect the lining of the gut and its microbiota. This leads to acute dysbiosis, which will alter your child's physiological (and psychological) functioning. Symptoms of poor gut health might include, but are not limited to, fatigue, headache, skin rashes, joint pain, abdominal pain, diarrhea or constipation, inability to focus, anxiety, depression, brain fog, poor dental health, and much more. An unhealthy gut also contributes to the late effects that up to 90 percent of pediatric cancer survivors experience.[1] These might include, but again are not limited to, poor bone health, cardiac problems, breathing problems, thyroid and other hormone-related issues, mental health challenges, and more.[2] Understanding cancer treatment's long-term effects on gut microbiota and psycho-physiological function is critical to improving survivors' physical and mental health.

The gut microbiota is an important modulator of metabolic, immune, psychological, and cognitive mechanisms. If we have an unhealthy gut, we are unhealthy. Unfortunately, there is currently no discussion in conventional oncology of the importance of the restoration of the gut microbiota after the completion of conventional treatment. Healing of the gut microbiota via targeted therapies could potentially prevent or reverse the psycho-physiological deficits often found in young survivors, ultimately leading to reduced symptom burden and improved health.[3]

The microbiome is an organ in its own right. It is composed of communities of bacteria, viruses, and fungi that have great complexity and develop from birth to approximately the age of three years old. Those first three years of life are crucial in supporting a developing microbiome. Vaginal birth and breastfeeding help build a healthy microbiome, whereas antibiotics before the age of three, cesarean births, and formula feeding can disrupt it. Studies show that children who are given antibiotics are more prone to chronic illnesses like eczema, asthma, IBD, and IBS.[4] What's more toxic to gut health than antibiotics? Cancer treatment. It is devastating to gut health and leaves lifelong lasting effects—unless the gut is healed.

The gut microbiota has many critical functions, including protection from pathogens, immune system development, and accessing the nutrients in food. Without healing a child's gut, the child will not be able to absorb nutrients from their food or supplements. They will not sustain a healthy immune system to protect from infections, and they will be vulnerable to inflammation that can contribute to relapse.

What Is a Leaky Gut?

The term *leaky gut* is used to describe a condition in which the intestines are hyperpermeable, meaning the intestinal lining has become excessively porous. As a result, undigested food molecules and waste flow into the bloodstream, where they do not belong. The body's reaction to such substances in the bloodstream can be dramatic. The liver is called in to screen out the particles that the intestinal lining was supposed to be managing, but the liver can't keep up. So these undigested food molecules, yeasts, and other pathogens begin to accumulate, causing immune and other physiological reactions.

The immune system starts to fight these invaders, going into full battle mode. Most often, a portion of these foreign bodies is absorbed into tissues throughout the body, causing the tissues to become inflamed. As an immune response, inflammation itself causes even more stress upon the system. As the body focuses on major battles, the little battles—like filtering the blood, reducing localized inflammation, targeting bacteria, regulating the gut—begin to be ignored. This can lead to an array of autoimmune conditions, which result from the body fighting itself. A cancer survivor might experience these autoimmune conditions as "late effects" from their treatment, but it might be helpful to consider whether the underlying cause, and therefore an appropriate response, might involve the health of the gut.

Why is this so important for cancer survivors? Because just *one* dose of chemotherapy can disrupt the microbiome so severely that it can take months, or even years, to heal. Despite the burgeoning awareness in the past two decades of the critical importance of the microbiome to human health, your child's gut health will not be addressed by your child's oncologist.

Your child's gut health won't even be addressed by most books about holistic cancer treatment.

Without healing intestinal hyperpermeability, the body cannot break down food into the nutrients your child needs to heal. You might be spending money and effort on quality "anticancer" supplements, but if your child's body is not capable of using these supplements because of a leaky gut and hyperactive immune response, your child is unlikely to experience much benefit. Worse, your child's immune system might be so busy with undigested food particles and other substances in the bloodstream to notice that cancer cells have started to emerge . . . again.

It took my daughter, Zuza, more than three years to heal her gut after five months of chemotherapy. That was three years of specific, gut-healing foods, herbs, and supplements, along with a major focus on sleep, movement, managing emotions, and avoiding toxic chemicals.

In fact, most of us are probably somewhere on the spectrum of mild to severe intestinal hyperpermeability. Why? Because intestinal permeability is also exacerbated by modern living: a diet full of refined sugar and processed foods, chronic stress, inflammation, over-the-counter medications, nutritional deficiencies such as zinc, and more.

Symptoms of a leaky gut can include multiple food sensitivities; brain fog; any autoimmune conditions; skin conditions such as acne, rashes, or eczema; inflammation symptoms such as allergies or dry eyes; GI symptoms such as diarrhea or constipation; irritable bowel disease; severe nutrient deficiencies; and small intestinal bacterial overgrowth. Causes include a history of chemotherapy or chemotherapy-like drugs used for irritable bowel disease (including Crohn's disease and ulcerative colitis) or rheumatoid arthritis and use of multiple antibiotics or steroids.

Because conventional cancer treatment can impact a child's baseline so dramatically, I don't test the gut health of a child unless they have been finished with treatment for at least three months. Instead, I recommend gut healing for all cancer patients (there isn't any downside, other than the time, effort, and some expense) and then conduct some testing when the time is right.

This testing might include conventional blood work covered by insurance, including C-reactive protein, LDH, sed rate, vitamin D3, vitamin B12, homocysteine, RBC zinc, and magnesium. While these lab tests do not measure intestinal permeability specifically, they offer clues about inflammation and nutritional deficiencies that might signal the extent of leaky gut—and at a relatively low cost. In my practice, I work with patients and their families to heal the gut for at least a year after conventional treatment ends before I order any additional in-depth testing.

For additional in-depth testing—again, when the time is right—there are three GI tests that I use:

The Cyrex Laboratories Array 2 Intestinal Antigenic Permeability Screen. This is a blood test that costs approximately $200 and must be ordered by a practitioner.

Organic Acid Test (OAT) by Mosaic Diagnostics (formerly Great Plains Laboratory). This is a urine test that costs approximately $100 and must be ordered by a practitioner. Turn-around time is approximately three to four weeks. It offers a metabolic snapshot of the patient's overall health, including markers for vitamin and mineral levels, as well as intestinal yeast and bacteria.

GI-MAP by Diagnostic Solutions Laboratory. This is a stool test that costs approximately $300 and must be ordered by a practitioner. Turn-around time is about four weeks. It uses quantitative polymerase chain reaction technology to detect parasites, bacteria, fungi, and more.

The Five Rs: Remove, Replace, Reinoculate, Repair, and Rebalance

How can we restore balance to the digestive system to restore health to the whole body? I have a protocol I like to use called the Five Rs: remove, replace, reinoculate, repair, and rebalance. Healing the gut is a multifactorial and individualized process, but in my opinion every patient will benefit from each of these five steps.

Remove

In order to heal your child's gut, you must remove things. This includes removing inflammatory foods from their diet, eliminating gut-harming medications such as antibiotics, and reducing the "bad bugs" that might be present in the gut already, such as bacteria or yeast, and that can be tackled with natural herbs and supplements.

Common inflammatory ingredients include nonorganic and GMO foods; artificial colors and flavors; refined sugars and high-fructose corn syrup;

nonorganic, nonsprouted bleached flours; gluten; soy; and corn. I recommend a nutrient-dense, low-carbohydrate, high-protein diet free of all of these ingredients. (See "Level 1 Nutrition" on page 189 for more details.)

In my experience, kids do best when they eliminate all grains, not just gluten. You can replace grains with organic millet, buckwheat, or quinoa, but continue to focus on fewer carbohydrates and more healthy fats, quality protein, probiotic-rich foods, and tons of vegetables.

For younger children up to eight years old who have yeast or other bacterial overgrowth, I often use Biocidin liposomal formula or liquid, based on weight. For older children, I recommend CandiBactin AR (one softgel one to three times per day) or CandiBactin BR (two tablets one to two times per day).

Replace

Replace digestive secretions by supplementing digestive enzymes and bile acids that are required for proper digestion and that may be compromised by diet or other factors. Additionally, you might want to add apple cider vinegar and bitters to your child's diet. I like Urban Moonshine bitters and Herb Pharm bittersweet, a few drops before meals. For digestive enzymes, I often use Ther-Biotic Vital-Zymes chewables and Enzymedica Kids Digest chewables.

Reinoculate

Help beneficial bacteria flourish with probiotic foods or supplements that contain the so-called "good" GI bacteria, such as *Bifidobacterium* and *Lactobacillus* species, and with prebiotics. Fermented foods and probiotic-rich foods include fermented veggies such as sauerkraut, yogurt, kimchi, miso, and beet kvass. Prebiotic foods include garlic, onions, leeks, sweet potatoes (cooked then cooled), and white potatoes (cooked then cooled).

In addition to these beneficial foods, I recommend quality probiotics, switching brands every three months to reinoculate the gut with different types of bacteria. Some brands I like are Ther-Biotic Baby, Ther-Biotic Children, Flourish, MetaKids Probiotic, HMF Child (chewables), Mega-SporeBiotic, Ther-Biotic Detox, and Ortho Biotic 100.

Repair

Help the lining of the GI tract repair itself by supplying key nutrients that are often depleted by disease, such as zinc, antioxidants, and the amino acid glutamine. Other supplements that can help repair the GI tract include omega-3 fatty acids, turmeric, vitamin A, vitamin C, ginger, and *Boswellia*. Demulcents can also contribute to GI tract repair. Sometimes referred to as mucoprotective or mucilage-producing agents, demulcents form a soothing film over the mucous membranes, relieving minor pain and inflammation. They can be taken in food, tea, powder, capsules, tinctures, or herbal preparations. Demulcent herbs include slippery elm, marshmallow, licorice, Oregon grape root, and aloe vera.

For severe gut issues, I make a gut-healing tea: Combine 1 teaspoon each of slippery elm bark, chopped marshmallow root, and chopped licorice root. Add 2 quarts of water to the herbs and soak for six to eight hours or overnight. In the morning, boil the mixture down to ½ quart and strain. Give your child 1 tablespoon of gut-healing tea every two hours.

A convenient way to get all these healing herbs is a blend of GI Revive (in pill or powder form), G.I. Fortify (pure encapsulations), SBI Protect or Intestinal Repair Complex, RF Plus, and Proflora 4R. Be aware, however, that these products can interfere with other supplement or medication absorption and with chemotherapies, so I highly recommend you work with a practitioner when choosing a gut-healing protocol. In addition to the above, some other products I like include Hemp Kids Oil and Ion Gut Support.

Finally, full-spectrum hemp oil deserves a note of its own because it can decrease intestinal permeability by helping to patch the holes in a leaky gut. Through regulating tight junction function, cannabinoids may help prevent food particles, infections, and other inflammatory agents from entering the bloodstream. This can reduce inflammation, preventing further damage to the gut wall.

Of course, repairing a leaky gut will rely heavily on food and nutrition. Some of the best foods for healing the gut include bone broth, whose collagen helps heal the stomach lining; healthy fats such as coconut oil, avocados, avocado oil, and ghee; and fermented foods such as sauerkraut, kefir, kimchi, beet kvass, and fermented vegetables like beets, cucumbers, and carrots.

Every meal should contain healthy fat, healthy protein, vegetables, and fermented foods. These foods can be tasty, and meals needn't be complicated. For example, breakfast might be eggs with spinach sautéed in coconut oil or ghee with a kefir smoothie or almond-flour pancakes with organic butter and bone broth to drink. Lunch might be a bone-broth based soup with quinoa or millet, chicken, and vegetables with a side of fermented beet salad. Dinner could be zucchini noodles with homemade pesto (garlic, walnuts, parsley, avocado oil) with avocado salad and a glass of beet kvass. For a snack, offer your child a green juice smoothie, organic nuts, a veggie plate with nut butter, or guacamole with grain-free chips. For dessert, indulge in a small square of 78 percent dark chocolate.

Rebalance

What does it mean to rebalance, especially in terms of healing the gut? Mostly it refers to lifestyle—how we live—and it might surprise you that I consider this even more important than diet and supplements. (That said, there *are* supplements that are very effective in reducing stress, including ashwagandha, full-spectrum hemp oil or CBD oil, licorice, holy basil, rhodiola root, and *Eleutherococcus* root.) Stress can prevent healing, even when we do everything else right. Stress can be exacerbated by poor sleep, lack of physical activity, and limited time outdoors. And it can definitely be exacerbated by a cancer diagnosis. So it's time to get serious—about being less serious. It's time to rebalance your life and help your child learn to rebalance theirs. This will not only help your child's gut heal; it will improve the well-being of your entire family.

Teach your kids to spend thirty minutes each day in activities they enjoy that help them unwind. There are a million activities that might fall into this category, but for example, you might include the following:

- Prayer or spiritual coloring books
- Meditation (I love the Insight Timer app or Headspace)
- Yoga
- Intentional breathing
- Reiki
- Drawing, painting, or sculpting
- Journaling
- Surfing or boogie boarding
- Participating in a support group

For a younger child, rebalance might include playing outside and taking an herbal bath before bed. A slightly older child might play outside, do some creative artwork or journaling, use an ashwagandha tincture and full-spectrum hemp oil, and take an herbal bath before bed. And a teenager might spend time outside; do yoga, breathwork, and meditate; and take holy basil and full-spectrum CBD oil or hemp tea before bed.

———

How long does it take to heal a child's gut after cancer treatment? It's impossible to say because every child starts from a different place and, for some children, the unhealthy gut is what contributed to the development of their cancer in the first place. Furthermore, conventional cancer treatment varies dramatically for each patient. The amount of time it takes to heal the gut depends on all of these variables, but a good rule of thumb is that it takes months to years to heal the gut. You can monitor your child's progress through symptoms and testing such as the OAT test.

For children who undergo bone marrow transplants, new studies suggest that fecal transplants may be beneficial for gut healing.[5] A clinical trial at Memorial Sloan Kettering Cancer Center has shown that fecal transplants can reestablish the good bacteria that is often lost in people who have had a bone marrow transplant for blood cancer. The trial collected the patient's own stool prior to the transplant and gave it back to the patient after the transplant to restore their microbiome.[6]

Small studies have also shown that fecal transplant can improve outcomes in graft-versus-host disease. A 2021 study showed that 82 percent of participants who had a fecal transplant after significant graft-versus-host-disease refractory (lack of response) to steroids improved.[7] Fecal transplants are also showing promise in the treatment of recurrent *Clostridioides difficile* (*C. diff*), a bacterial infection common in pediatric cancer patients, as well as in patients who are not responding to immunotherapy drugs.[8]

CHAPTER 12

Heal the Child, Heal the Family

I CALL IT A BEAUTIFUL SHATTERING. PEDIATRIC CANCER WILL SHATTER you, your child, your relationships, your partner, and your other children. This is unavoidable. Shattering is part of the process. So is putting yourself back together.

Why do I refer to it as beautiful? As painful as it is, you have also been presented with an opportunity to take your shattered self and put yourself back together in a new way—leaving now unnecessary pieces behind. Cancer will change your perspective and values. There will be pieces of yourself that no longer serve you. You will be changed, and you can use this opportunity to change into a more authentic version of yourself. More importantly, you have the opportunity to model this journey in a healthy way for your child. It will be painful for them, too. It can also be beautiful.

Your partner will also be changed, and this may challenge your marriage. Your other children will be changed, and this will impact your relationship with them. Every person in your family is going to change as a result of this experience. Your family dynamics will change and your relationships with the outside world will change. You will be building your life and your family's life again, this time with the insights of pain and suffering as your tools.

From my experience, tension can build right away between you and your partner. It is important to remember you're on the same team and your goal is the same—to help your child survive. Contrary to what you might think, parents of a child with cancer do not experience a higher risk of divorce.[1]

Remember that your partner might process and respond to grief, fear, stress, and trauma in a different way than you do. Your partner might also have different opinions than you do about the role, if any, of integrative support versus conventional care. Additionally, tension can sometimes start months to years later, when things are supposed to be OK. In addition to all the strategies for self-care—such as good nutrition, movement, and integrative support for stress management and well-being—marriages can benefit from talk therapy, setting aside time for one another, and fierce compassion for each other and yourself—even if, and maybe especially when, you disagree. Having a child with cancer will impact your marriage, but bear in mind that it's possible to become stronger together.

If you have other children, you already know that they will be impacted by their sibling's cancer diagnosis and treatment. Regardless of what age they are, this experience will impact them—and it might impact them in unexpected or uncomfortable ways. For example, they might act out in jealousy and then feel guilty about it, because your child with cancer will be getting so much attention. They might feel angry that their sibling's needs are often put first and their sibling's pain gets more attention. Up to 63 percent of siblings of a cancer patient will experience significant challenges adjusting to the cancer diagnosis.[2] Siblings of children with cancer experience more depression, more anxiety, and worse peer relationships, sometimes even years after their sibling completes treatment.

What's the answer to this? As you might expect by now, there isn't an easy one. But you might start by acknowledging and trying to understand how your child's cancer diagnosis and treatment is affecting your other children, even if they don't talk about it much. Be careful not to project your own feelings and fears onto them. Any time they want to talk, listen. Children can read the energy of the home and the energy of a given situation. Honesty is important because a child's imagination can be far scarier than reality, but it's also important to speak with care and not underestimate the impact information will have. Give your children lots of healthy outlets for their emotions. I tried to keep my son involved in outdoor programs, which helped him immensely. Your other children might (or might not) want to make positive lifestyle changes alongside their sibling, as a way to feel that you are caring as much for them. It's complicated, and it's different for everyone and every family. As a caregiver, your job is to model compassion, forgiveness, resilience, and imperfection in difficult circumstances, which in itself is a loving example to set for your children.

Psychoneuroimmunology

Psychoneuroimmunology is the study of how the immune system and the central nervous system interact. Childhood cancer has physical, neurological, and psychosocial effects. This results in chronic stress, which increases disease risk. We know that chronic stress makes us more susceptible to everything from the common cold to cancer. A 2019 nonrandomized, open-label clinical trial assessed whether a psychoneuroimmunology-based intervention would enhance immunity in children with acute lymphoblastic leukemia undergoing chemotherapy. Researchers found an increase in immunity markers along with a decrease in use of antibiotics, antipyretics, analgesics, and respiratory therapy. In other words, psychoneuroimmunology-based interventions increased patient well-being.[3]

The stress that your child experiences during treatment affects their body to such an extent that it may impact their response to treatment and affect their immune system. This is to say: Quality of life matters. Even if your child's oncology team does not understand the clinical implications of programs supporting positive coping behaviors, you have a lot of power as a parent to implement psychological, social, and physical activities that will support your child during and after treatment.

Supportive psychological, social, and physical activities will also be important for your other children, your spouse, and yourself. Many parents will stop taking care of themselves completely when they have a child fighting cancer. This is devastating, because as the caregiver, your child depends on your well-being. When I was in the hospital with my daughter, Zuza, I tried to work out every day, ate well, prioritized sleep, and meditated. I took care of myself for me and for her. It's easy to tell yourself that you'll take care of yourself once your child is OK, but your child's journey will be lifelong. Do not wait for the day when things are finally OK. Things will start to become OK when you start to also take care of yourself.

Hypothalamic-Pituitary-Adrenal (HPA) Axis Dysfunction

The moment we hear the words that our child has cancer our body experiences an acute stress response, also known as fight-or-flight. For many parents, that first month is a blur. In response to the stress, our bodies release epinephrine and cortisol, and we live on this energy for months. We are in survival mode.

We are thrown into a foreign world of chemotherapy, radiation, new terminology, and the idea that our child may die. We have to sign paperwork allowing potentially life-threatening side effects. We have to balance the needs of our terrified child, and their terrified siblings, and our distraught partner—with things that suddenly seem insignificant, like our job or petty disputes. The stress hormones keep us going. We need them in order to do what needs to be done. But at some point, they begin to wear us down.

Survival mode can last months or even years. It might come and go through relapses or long periods of treatment. Children who have entered remission may be sent home with little follow-up or support. Friends and family members might be celebrating that "your child is fine now." But you wonder: Why do you now feel even more terrible than you did while you were running on adrenaline for all those weeks and months?

Believe it or not, the first six months after treatment has ended can be even harder than treatment itself. During this time, you might realize that your old life is never coming back. The fantasy of a return to your old life may have been sustaining you through weeks and months of your child's treatment. You may have found yourself dreaming of simple joys (and now petty-seeming problems) you once took for granted: the mundane routine of your job, the impossible balancing act of parenthood in the twenty-first century. Whatever your life was before your child was diagnosed with cancer is over. I don't mean you won't have vacations and birthday parties and trivial problems. I mean it will all be different. You can't unsee what you've now seen. You can't undo what your child has been through. It changes everything, and there is no going back.

There's something else: Your new normal will take a lot of work to build. Your family has just experienced so much trauma. The outside world wants you to go back to the family they used to know. Your friendships will change and you will change. Many of your relationships, including with your children and partner, will require a rebuilding or renegotiation. In my opinion, it's better to accept this than fight against it. It will be hard—at times even excruciating. It is also an opportunity to build anew, with the wisdom you have gained and the values you now hold.

Except there's more. You will likely be doing all this rebuilding in a state of post-traumatic hypothalamic-pituitary-adrenal (HPA) axis dysfunction. While a fight-or-flight response is essential in survival situations, we weren't designed to live in this state on a chronic basis. And you, your child, and your family probably have been. Once you are home and things are supposed to be normal, you might be continuing to release those hormones through constant worry and vigilance about your child relapsing, or your sympathetic (fight or flight) and parasympathetic (rest and digest) nervous systems may have become completely dysfunctional, affecting all aspects of your physiology and psychology. It is likely that every member of your family will have to heal HPA axis dysfunction.

What contributes to HPA axis dysfunction? In addition to chronic stress (whether perceived or real), a lot of things can contribute to it. This is actually good news, because it means that while you can't control the circumstances of your life, you can exercise a measure of control over how you respond to them. Things that contribute to HPA axis dysfunction include disruptions to circadian rhythm, inadequate or poor sleep, poor diet, blood sugar dysregulation, chronic inflammation, and environmental toxins.

Of course, it's not as easy as it sounds to mitigate these circumstances. For example, it's hard to maintain healthy sleeping patterns when you're anxiously waiting for test results or sleeping in a hospital room chair while your child undergoes inpatient chemotherapy treatment or a bone marrow transplant. When you haven't slept well, you're less likely to eat well, and when you aren't eating well, it becomes harder to motivate yourself to exercise, even just a little.

I'm not saying any of this is easy. I'm saying that the little things can make a huge difference. A little daily movement is better than none. A few yoga poses, a little stretching, a short walk outside—all of these can help. What's more, they can begin to create a positive feedback loop. That short walk helps you feel better, which makes you want to eat organic vegetables instead of pizza, and that helps you sleep better at night. The small moments and the small interventions matter, for you, your child, and your family. Don't overlook these opportunities or discount the impact they can have on your life.

In addition to lifestyle modifications, you might consider incorporating adaptogens, which are a class of herbs that help the body cope with stress. Adaptogens include ashwagandha and nervines such as St. John's wort, lavender, and chamomile. Certain medicinal mushrooms have healing properties. And vitamins such as vitamin C, B-complex, and L-theanine can play a role in stress management.

Addiction

You might be surprised to see a section about addiction in a book on child-hood cancer. Addiction is more relevant than you might imagine. There are pronounced risks for both your child and you. In terms of your child, my feeling is this: There is a place for pain medication in pediatric cancer, but it's important not to overuse it. Studies demonstrate a link between opioids and cancer growth.[4] Certain cancer cells have five to ten times as many opioid receptors as noncancerous cells. Opioids can increase proliferation, mitigation, and invasion of tumor cells.[5]

Morphine is regularly used for children undergoing bone marrow biopsy. In my opinion, it's not usually necessary. Some full-spectrum CBD oil may help with discomfort. If a child must undergo a painful surgery, it is impera-tive to wean them off opioids as soon as possible. Ibuprofen and, even better, full-spectrum hemp oil or cannabis oil (depending on its legality where you are) can get you far. Heat packs and cool packs can also help, as do certain essential oils and pulsed electromagnetic field (PEMF) devices.

Addiction among caregivers is also not uncommon. This can be alcohol or drug addiction, or it can be food or disease addiction. While an occasional glass of wine at the end of a hard day can be OK, watch yourself, because it can easily spiral into a habit. Use breathing techniques, time in nature, and exercise to manage those hard days. Turn to prayer, meditation, and full-spectrum hemp oil for your anxieties. Make a list of the coping mecha-nisms that work best for you and use them.

Long-Term Healing

The foundation of long-term healing is going to be the same as day-to-day acute stress management: nutrient-dense food, daily movement, self-care rou-tines, and good sleep habits. Watch for addictive behaviors and make the effort to engage in and model healthy, clear, and compassionate communication.

There are many different ways of approaching a self-care routine and heal-ing. A lot of what I cover here has been touched on in other chapters. But once your child is through treatment, I think it's worth considering it through a different lens. You are no longer trying to sustain your child, yourself, and your family through the intensely acute experience of treatment. You are now devoting yourself in a new way to recovery—body, mind, spirit—of your child, their siblings, you, your marriage, and your family as a unit. You may not be married, you may not have other children, and—for some of you—you may be experiencing the heartbreak, not of recovery, but of your child's death. Everybody's experience will be different. My point is that some deep healing from deep trauma—far more than I can cover in this chapter; this chapter is just the beginning—is in order. Please take it seriously. Every day give yourself time, space, and permission to engage in the healing process.

Meditation

Studies show that meditation is a complementary approach in the treatment of post-traumatic stress disorder (PTSD), anxiety, and depression for adults.[6] Meditation can also help children.[7] It is best to incorporate regular meditation into children's lives when they are young. My children are home-schooled, and meditation followed by prayer is something we do every day as part of their education.

I also like to wind down the day with my kids with meditation (and some red-light therapy) most evenings. Phone apps like Calm and InsightTimer give access to thousands of meditations. Finding a meditation teacher or app that you and your children connect with is important. Our family loves Sarah Blondin and Dr. Joe Dispenza.

Breathwork

Trauma can be expelled through breathwork by releasing tension and energy that is deeply rooted within the subconsciousness. Studies demonstrate that breathing-based meditations diminish trauma. One helpful form of breathing is alternate nostril breathing. Studies demonstrate that deep breathing can lessen anxiety in kids.[8]

Cognitive-Behavioral Therapy

Cognitive-behavioral therapy has been demonstrated to be an effective form of therapy for PTSD, anxiety, and depression for both kids and adults. Play therapy is often most appropriate for younger children, whereas older children and adults may benefit from talk therapy.

ART and EMDR

Accelerated resolution therapy (ART) and eye movement desensitization and reprocessing (EMDR) are similar approaches that alleviate suffering from trauma, PTSD, anxiety, and depression. ART therapists guide the client to voluntarily replace traumatic images in the mind with positive images, primarily through the use of specific eye movements that produce theta waves in the brain connected to creativity, daydreaming, and intuition. A special aspect of ART therapy is that the client does not necessarily need to *talk* about the details of the trauma. Incredible progress can sometimes be made in the time frame of a single session.

EMDR is similar to ART in that it uses specific eye movements to reprocess memories associated with a traumatic experience, thereby desensitizing the brain to the traumatic memory (as opposed to replacing it, in ART).

Reiki and Energy Healing

Reiki is a Japanese form of energetic bodywork that can help manage stress and promote healing. In a recent study published in *Military Medicine*, researchers observed a significant drop in PTSD symptoms following Reiki practice.[9] Another study measured the effect of Reiki for managing pain in pediatric cancer patients undergoing inpatient stem cell transplant and found that those patients who received Reiki were better able to manage their pain.[10]

Nature Therapy

We don't give nature enough credit! Get your family outside. Kids heal in nature, and so do adults. Sign your kids up for an outdoor program and get them outside after school or on the weekends all year round. Bundle yourself up when it's cold outside and take a daily walk, no matter the weather. Studies demonstrate that forest bathing helps alleviate depression and anxiety and can even enhance immunity.[11]

Adaptogens

Adaptogens are herbs (and fungi) that help our body deal with stress. These plants and their active extracts support adrenal function, reduce fatigue, and build endurance. They help us adapt to stress and restore our capacity to cope and respond. In multiple studies, ashwagandha has been associated with a significant reduction in anxiety and depression.[12] It is safe for use in children, though it often takes a few weeks to notice the effect. In addition to ashwagandha, some common adaptogens include the following:

- American ginseng is well known for its ability to increase physical strength and stamina. It also supports a healthy memory and mental acuity. It will help to relieve exhaustion and improve mental alertness and memory.

- Eleuthero root improves normal mental clarity and emotional stamina during stressful situations, improves physical endurance, and supports healthy immune system functioning.
- Holy basil helps restore vitality and promote overall health, allowing a gentler response to stress.
- Rhodiola supports healthy immune system functioning.
- Schisandra berries aid with concentration, coordination, and endurance. Schisandra is known to calm the heart and mind.
- Cordyceps is a mushroom that has long been used in traditional Chinese medicine for immune support.

Nervines

Nervines are herbs that nourish and support the central nervous system to rebalance and restore restfulness in the body.[13] They are similar to adaptogens (and you can take them in combination with adaptogens) but are more targeted to restoring restfulness to the body (adaptogens are more specifically targeted for stress). Some common nervines include the following:

- Chamomile can be helpful for relieving mild daily mental stress.
- Lavender is a calming herb often used in aromatherapy for its mild calming action.
- Lemon balm helps with nervous exhaustion, gloom, and restlessness. (It also smells amazing.)
- Passionflower relieves tension and nervous restlessness and supports restful sleep.
- Skullcap is gentle and nourishing to the nervous system. It relieves occasional tension and stress, ruminating thoughts, and nervousness. It can be used as needed during stressful situations or at night before bed.
- Valerian is a potent herb that supports relaxation. It is stronger than some other nervines. Be aware that in some people it can cause stimulation. In this case, switch to a different nervine.

Infrared Sauna

I discussed the amazing benefits of sauna for detoxification in chapter 10, but research also demonstrates that infrared sauna is an effective tool for treating depression and anxiety.[14] The effect can last as long as six weeks after a single sauna treatment.[15]

CBD and Full-Spectrum Hemp Oil

The human body's endocannabinoid system is like a conductor sending signals to endocannabinoid receptors throughout the body, including those in the brain, heart, endocrine system, connective tissues, glands, and immune cells. This is one reason endocannabinoids can alleviate so many different types of symptoms. Regular use of a quality full-spectrum hemp oil can reduce anxiety and help kids and adults settle down before sleep. Dosing for sleep and anxiety is highly individualized; it can start at 10 milligrams per day and go up to 300 milligrams in some situations.

The hemp plant contains over a hundred cannabinoids; the most studied one is CBD. This plant should be full spectrum. Full-spectrum hemp oil does contain THC, but in minimal amounts—enough to be effective, but not enough to cause any psychoactive side effects. Be smart about your sourcing and ask lots of questions. You want hemp from a supplier you trust, from plants that have not been treated with herbicides or pesticides.

Psychedelics

Drugs used for psychedelic therapy can include LSD, psilocybin, DMT, mescaline, and MDMA. A 2020 review of twenty-four studies on the use of psychedelic drugs to treat anxiety reported a 65 percent reduction in anxiety symptoms.[16] Another study found that psilocybin may be as effective as selective serotonin reuptake inhibitors for treating depression.[17] The use of psychedelics is illegal in many places. In the United States, you can explore participating in clinical trials, or, if you are willing to travel outside the United States, look for a reputable retreat center.

Many people use psychedelics by *microdosing*, which refers to taking extremely small doses for psychological benefits, without the psychoactive effects. Studies demonstrate a reduction in depression and anxiety even at microdoses.[18] To be completely clear, I do not recommend psychedelics—in any dose—for children.

Pharmaceuticals

In my opinion, medications for depression, anxiety, and PTSD have their place and can be helpful in the short term, but I consider these a last resort, something that can get you stable enough to think clearly and manage your life, so you have the bandwidth to explore other therapies, improve your nutrition, get the sleep you need, and invest in safer, more long-term strategies for self-care.

The FDA has recently approved a nasal spray derived from ketamine for depression. In one study, 70 percent of patients with treatment-resistant depression who were started on the intranasal ketamine spray and oral antidepressant improved.[19]

Palliative Care

In my role as an integrative practitioner, I have been part of many families' decisions to move a child to palliative care. Palliative care is a compassionate approach to the end of the journey, aimed at enhancing quality of life and providing relief from the physical, emotional, and psychological suffering a patient may be facing. Unlike curative treatments, palliative care focuses on alleviating pain and symptoms, managing side effects, and addressing the unique needs of both the child and the family. There are palliative care specialists who work collaboratively with medical teams to ensure comfort and self-determination for the patient. Palliative care is a way for a patient and their family to be home together for those precious final days without the sounds and smells of a hospital, in the comfort of their own bed, with their belongings and loved ones.

The decision to move to palliative care is, of course, one the hardest decisions a family will ever make. It usually comes when the chances of a cure become so low, and the treatment so toxic, that a child's quality of life is severely compromised. Sometimes children—usually older children—will come to this junction on their own, when they have simply had enough of it all, and reach a point of persuading their parents that they need to be done with treatment.

In Zuza's case, we have been given the option of palliative care for a long time. From the perspective of conventional oncologists, her chances for a cure are small enough that we are always presented with the option of refusing conventional treatment. But a very determined Zuza has always been clear with us: She's not done pursuing a cure. If a child is old enough to be part of the conversation, they need to be. In our case, Zuza has always answered the question for us.

For many families, it's not so clear. Many parents will, naturally, struggle over whether to encourage their child to keep fighting or to support the decision to lay down the sword. Parenting is full of decisions, many of them difficult, and in my mind there is no question: This is the most difficult decision any parent—or child, or family—will ever have to make. Pause for a moment and let that soak in. If you're struggling, that would be appropriate. If you're in despair, that would be appropriate. If you feel that you are going through something that very few people will ever understand, you are correct.

We don't want to rob our children of their lives, their future, their opportunities, their experiences, their destiny. We also don't want to force them into needless suffering, especially if there is no realistic possibility of an acceptable quality of life. I don't have those answers. I wish I did. But there are a few thoughts I would like to share.

One of the hardest questions is when. I want you to know that there is no perfect answer to this question. It is incredibly individualized and nuanced, because every child and every family is different. There may be religious, cultural, and personal factors at play. And, of course, nobody can predict the future. Nobody can tell you what decision will lead you to the most joy and the least suffering. This decision relies on information, instinct, and deep listening—to your child, your other family members, perhaps God, or your own inner compass. It is important to know that palliative care is not a one-way street. You can return to curative care.

I also want to discuss what an integrative approach to palliative care might look like. There may be situations where you might still want to employ certain integrative techniques for quality-of-life and wellness benefits. Sometimes even the most holistically oriented family will choose conventional pain management approaches, since long-term effects are not a concern at this stage. In terms of nutrition, many children will be on a feeding tube at this point, but if they're able to eat, should you make them their favorite comfort foods? These decisions have no correct answer other than to follow your gut and your child's wants and needs.

To the families who have walked this path and held their child's hand as they passed away—or to those who are facing this—I want you to know that I am wowed by your bravery. You are somehow still here breathing and still living, and you deserve immense compassion and credit, no matter what has happened along the way. I send you love and light.

––––––––

I have written an entire book discussing how to support a child who has or had cancer with nutrition, supplements, therapies, and detoxification. I'm here to tell you that emotional healing is equally, if not more, important. The moment your child is diagnosed with cancer will change everything. Do not underestimate what you, your child, and your family have endured and continue to endure. Give yourself compassion and credit for making it this far.

It is my hope that the information in this book has helped you, your child, and your family heal. But the truth is that having a seriously ill child is a terrifying journey into the unknown with no guarantees. (Of course, life never has any guarantees—for anyone.) Even though I have been on this journey for a long time, I don't have all the answers for you. I wish I did. I wish I were farther down my own path so I could tell you how to do it—or even tell you with complete confidence that it can be done. The truth is, after years of supporting my daughter, Zuza, through multiple relapses, there are days when I wonder if this heavy feeling on my chest will ever go away. I wonder how it will all turn out.

But what I do know is that from the beginning, you will need to make many difficult decisions, have many difficult conversions, and entertain many difficult thoughts in your own heart and mind. You will need to decide how you want to walk this path and who will be walking it with you. Do not give your intuitive power away. Listen to the experts; they have been here before, they know their field, and they can guide you. But don't abdicate your authority to them. You are the person who is ultimately responsible for your child. Accept the information and advice from experts with gratitude. And then take full responsibility and make the best decisions you can.

As you, I hope, have learned, there is no magic bullet. But I believe that there is a better way than what conventional treatment alone has to offer. You can use nutrition and nutraceuticals to protect your child's healthy cells while making chemotherapy, immunotherapy, or radiation more effective. You can use gentler alternatives to pharmaceuticals to address the many side effects your child will experience. You can dramatically reduce side effects during treatment through metabolic therapies. You can heal your child's gut, help their body detoxify, and reduce the odds of late effects and complications. My hope is that you can even contribute to remission and reduce the chance of relapse.

Equally importantly, you can also learn to step into the trauma and find ways to breathe and center yourself and even through pain and chaos to find your breath and the source of life. You can be patient with yourself and know that healing as a family is a lifelong journey and that the new normal can be more beautiful, more meaningful, and more fulfilling.

Your child deserves a comprehensive approach to healing. Leave no rock unturned. I know it's not easy, but it can be better. There is a better way.

Epilogue

As I contemplate the words I'm about to share with you, my heart beats fast as I think back over our family's journey. It began with Zuza's initial diagnosis eight years ago and then her relapse three years ago following a five-year period of remission. Since her first relapse, our family has embarked on an extraordinary voyage, encompassing two bone marrow transplants, participation in medical trials, countless weeks of nerve-racking anticipation for test results, moments of celebrating the news, and moments of screaming inside. Our journey has been a mosaic of moments—sometimes sad and often hard—but through it all our journey has been beautiful and full of memories and laughter.

Our medical treatments have taken us from St. Louis to Chicago, with Houston on the horizon. Along the way, we've made memories exploring new cities, restaurants, and adapting to different homes. We've basked in the warmth of the sun during extended stays in Florida and Mexico, finding solace in the simple joys of life.

What has become evident to me is that we are not merely enduring this journey, we are actively *living* through it. We are navigating the difficult terrain, the kind that inflicts unbearable pain, and simultaneously, we are savoring the beautiful moments—the simple pleasures of togetherness and the privilege of watching Zuza grow into a preteen. In the face of these trials, my most valuable advice is not medical or integrative but rather a profound philosophy of living through it.

I encourage you to breathe through the hardships. Embrace the complexity of life, with its challenges and joys, and remember that it is the act of living through it that truly defines our resilience and spirit.

Currently, Zuza is home, recovering from an infection. In a few more weeks, as a family, we will be heading to Houston for a trial. This trial, known as CAR T, represents a form of immunotherapy that we hope will induce full remission for Zuza. Instead of the conventional approach involving chemotherapy, our local medical team is opting for a different method to achieve remission this time, with the hope that this approach will allow for her third transplant to "stick." Yes, if CAR T proves suc-cessful in achieving remission, our next step will be a third transplant. This marks our best and perhaps only chance at a cure, albeit one that is rare and carries inherent risks. A third transplant isn't often done, and it's a daunting prospect but one we are prepared for. I have the tools to take her through CAR T and another transplant, and Zuza has the will to keep trying. Throughout it all, we are bound together by one powerful force: HOPE.

My local medical team frequently emphasizes that for children with AML, a fortunate few may achieve a cure, while the less fortunate face a harsh reality of living for just one to two years. What's remarkable, and even unprecedented in the experience of our conventional oncologists, is that we've been alongside Zuza's AML journey for over eight years. Not one of our conventional oncology doctors has ever taken care of a patient with AML for eight-plus years. They attribute this to the integrative support we've provided for Zuza. I believe that they are beginning to realize that this inte-grative approach truly does offer a better way.

I wish I could assure you that this "better way" guarantees sustained remis-sion and a complete absence of side effects, but cancer journeys, like Zuza's, are often marked by their unpredictability and heartbreaking moments. Yet I can unequivocally state that our choice to pursue a holistic approach, our decisions to decline certain medications, and the unique strategies we've adopted are the very reasons Zuza stands here today, prepared to embrace her potentially final and curative treatment.

Zuza's resilience and our collective determination have steered us through the intricacies of her battle against AML, and in the process, they have illumi-nated the potential of a different path—a better path—filled with hope and, above all, the unwavering belief in a brighter, healthier future.

My second piece of advice is to nurture your relationships and be gentle with one another throughout this challenging journey. The strain of dealing with a serious illness can place a tremendous burden on family bonds. It tests the foundations of your marriage, if you have one. Although it may seem counterintuitive, I can confidently say that my own marriage is now stronger than ever. While it may be heart-wrenching for your other children, I firmly believe that this experience will mold my son into a more compassionate and beautiful human being.

This path is arduous on the body, so remember to care for yours, nourish it, and show it love. It can be equally demanding on the spirit, so allocate time for self-care, infusing your spirit with love and strength. Additionally, the journey is taxing on the mind, often spiraling it into a vortex of anxious thoughts. Remind yourself that your mind is not in charge, and urge it to stop weaving so many distressing narratives.

In the midst of all these trials, Zuza and Fin have embarked on an online school journey with Valor, which they genuinely enjoy. This development has lightened the load of homeschooling for me, allowing me to create a course tailored to pediatric cancer patients. Meanwhile, my husband has joined my medical practice to enhance patient care and workflow, enabling me to dedicate the majority of my professional time to caring for oncology patients.

Amid the whirlwind of this challenging journey, I found the inspiration to write a book. My hope is that this book makes essential information more accessible for everyone. This possibility brings me a deep sense of peace and fulfillment.

Acknowledgments

To my beloved daughter, Zuza: You are the reason for this book. The moment of your diagnosis marked a profound turning point in my life. I changed my career, I changed myself, and I made a promise to support families like ours on this journey. Every day, I make it my mission to learn more, to unearth better ways of providing the support you and other beautiful babies like you deserve.

Your diagnosis forced me to confront my own fears, to navigate through the tears, and to discover how to truly embrace life, even when it's uncomfortable, even when it's unpredictable. You, my Zuza, are nothing short of extraordinary, and I know this more deeply than anyone else. I know that we often chuckle when people refer to you as a "warrior"—it's a cliché often thrown at cancer patients. But I've witnessed the magnitude of your suffering, not all of which was physical, and yet you recover with such grace, and you continually give the human experience another chance. I love you—I can practically see you rolling those eyes at me as I write this, and I sense your slight smile because I always get so emotional. I adore you.

To my dear husband, who has been steadfastly walking alongside me on this journey—*living through it*—I want to express my gratitude for the love you've showered abundantly upon our kids and for filling our world with so much laughter and joy, even during the most trying times. Thank you for believing with me. Thank you for those moments where I could only muster 10 percent . . . Because you always provided the other 90 percent.

To my sweet son, Fin—this journey we speak of is what you call life; it is all you have ever known. Thank you for being an incredible brother to Zuza. Your love, your affection, and the comforting hugs you offer her have been a balm to her worries and a demonstration of pure sibling love. The way in which you bring such immense comfort and joy to us all is a testament to the beautiful soul that you are.

Thank you to my mom. You are the embodiment of the very best version of a mom that I could ever dream of. Your endless supply of hugs, the nourishing bone broths, and the nutritious food runs to the hospital have been my source of comfort and strength. Your unwavering love and support have been a bedrock for me to lean on. To my dad: Thank you for your calming presence and words, and the way you always say, "It will be OK, you'll see." You never, ever make us feel like you don't want to make all those runs to the pharmacies, grocery stores, and all the other places we dream up on an almost daily basis. Thank you. I could not have done any of this without you both.

To my mentor, Dr. Nasha Winters, thank you for walking through Zuza's first transplant with me—for supporting me in my depths and teaching me to have more guts. Thank you for being the flame carrier for this metabolic approach to cancer.

To the sweetest and smartest man I am humbled to text and sometimes even speak with: Dr. Paul Anderson. Your virtual care of my Zuza and your help making so many decisions that I would have otherwise been making on my own has made me one of your biggest fans (I know you have many). Our family adores you.

To my fellow cancer mama Laetitia—thank you for help on all of this. And to my editor, Brianne—this book literally would not have seen the world without all your hard work and above and beyond dedication—for that, I thank you.

To my dear friend Ellen—you have watched over me for all these years and created a space for us to swear and cry—thank you.

To my patients—thank you for the amazing things you have taught me, thank you to so many fellow cancer mamas for allowing me to hold you and holding me back. Thank you for the trust and patience you have given me in knowing that I am also on this journey.

Interpreting Test Results

THIS APPENDIX OFFERS INFORMATION ON HOW TO INTERPRET THE TEST results covered in chapter 3. I want to stress that it is the responsibility of your child's oncology team and integrative practitioner to interpret the test results, not yours. However, as you know by now, I encourage parents to gain a deeper understanding and be well informed about their child's condition. When using this resource, please remember never to become fixated on a single abnormal value. Instead, focus on the broader patterns of the laboratory results. If you encounter an abnormal value that seems out of place or inconsistent, recheck the lab before drawing any conclusions or taking action. Use this appendix as a tool to facilitate discussions with your medical team, ask questions, and explore your child's health. It is not meant for self-diagnosis.

Please also note that I have attempted to provide the most suitable reference ranges for pediatric patients. However, be aware that different units of measurement may be used for the results you receive. Always ensure that your test results and this appendix share the same units. If they don't match, you can find online calculators to help with conversions. Remember that the reference ranges for your child's specific lab results may differ. This appendix serves as a general guideline and should not replace the expert guidance provided by your integrative practitioner and oncologist.

Complete Blood Count (CBC)

As described in chapter 3, the CBC measures the different types of cells found in the blood—both mature and immature red blood cells and different types of white blood cells such as lymphocytes and neutrophils—as well as platelets (cell fragments) and hemoglobin (a protein that carries oxygen to the cells). The CBC measures complete count by volume, as cells per liter, grams per deciliter (dL, one-tenth of a liter), microliter per cubic milliliter (m3, one-billionth of a liter per mm3), or femtoliter (fL, one-quadrillionth of a liter). The CBC also measures ratios, such as concentration of hemoglobin, for example, and neutrophil to lymphocyte ratios.

CBC Measurements of Red Blood Cells

Red Blood Cell Count (RBC) ($'10\wedge6$/uL) measures the total number of red blood cells in the blood.

Reference range (RR): 4.1–5.3 $'10\wedge6$/uL

Above RR can indicate: Dehydration, stress, respiratory distress, vitamin C need, myeloproliferative disease

Below RR can indicate: Anemia, vitamin B12 deficiency, internal bleeding, liver and/or kidney dysfunction

Hematocrit (L/L) (%) measures the volume percentage of red blood cells in the blood.

RR: 35–45%

Above RR can indicate: Asthma, dehydration, diarrhea

Below RR can indicate: Anemia, digestive inflammation, vitamin C deficiency

Reticulocyte Count (RC) (%) measures the total number of reticulocytes (immature red blood cells) in the blood as a percentage of total red blood cells.

RR: 0.5–3.0% of total RBC

Above RR can indicate: Anemia (such as following treatment for anemia or following a bone marrow transplant), microscopic internal bleeding

Below RR can indicate: Anemia, adrenal hypofunction, bone marrow failure, response to pharmaceutical drugs (antivirals), response to anticancer therapy

Mean Corpuscular Volume (MCV) (fL) measures the size of red blood cells.

RR: 82.0–89.9 fL

Above RR can indicate: Anemia, vitamin B12 or folate deficiency, hypochlorhydria (stomach acid deficiency), vitamin C deficiency

Below RR can indicate: Iron deficiency/anemia, vitamin B6 deficiency, internal bleeding, heavy metal burden, digestive inflammation, intestinal parasites

Hemoglobin (g/dL) is a protein in red blood cells that carries oxygen.

RR: 9.5–17 g/dL, but dependent on age

Above RR can indicate: Asthma, dehydration, diarrhea

Below RR can indicate: Anemia, vitamin C deficiency, digestive inflammation, internal bleeding, response to chemotherapy

Mean Corpuscular Hemoglobin (MCH) (pg) measures the amount of hemoglobin in the blood and can be helpful in determining the type of anemia.

RR: 28.0–31.0 pg

Above RR can indicate: Anemia, hypochlorhydria (stomach acid deficiency)

Below RR can indicate: Anemia, internal bleeding, heavy metal burden, vitamin C deficiency

Mean Corpuscular Hemoglobin Concentration (MCHC) (%) or can be reported as (g/dL) measures the concentration of hemoglobin in red blood cells.

RR: 32–35% of total RBC

Above RR can indicate: Anemia, hypochlorhydria

Below RR can indicate: Vitamin C deficiency, heavy metal burden

Red Cell Distribution Width (RDW) (%) measures the difference in volume and size of red blood cells. It can be helpful in understanding hematological disorders and monitoring the effects of anticancer therapy.

RR: 11.7–15.0% of total RBC

Above RR can indicate: Iron deficiency/anemia, vitamin B12 or folate deficiency, recovering bone marrow post-transplant, post RBC transfusion

Below RR can indicate: Post-hemorrhagic anemia

CMC of White Blood Cells

White Blood Cell Count (WBC) ('10^3/uL) measures the total number of white blood cells in the blood.

Reference range (RR): 3.7–11.0 '10^3/uL

Above RR can indicate: Acute viral infection, acute bacterial infection, stress, presence of certain cancers including leukemia

Below RR can indicate: Chronic infection (including viral, Lyme, mold), chronic bacterial infection, suppressed by anticancer treatment like chemotherapy or radiation, indication of certain cancers like leukemia

Neutrophils (% and ´10^3/uL) are white blood cells used by the body to combat bacterial or pyrogenic infections.

    RR: 40–60% of total WBC

    Above RR can indicate: Viral or bacterial infection, inflammation

    Below RR can indicate: Blood disease including anemia and leukemia, chronic viral infection, adrenal dysfunction, intestinal parasites, recovering bone marrow

Bands (%) are immature neutrophils.

    RR: <5% of total WBC

    Above RR can indicate: Recovering bone marrow (post-transplant), infection

Lymphocytes (% and 10^3/uL) are a type of white blood cell that help the body fight disease and infection.

    RR: 24–44% of total WBC

    Above RR can indicate: Viral disease, viral infections, infectious mononucleosis, bacterial infections, inflammation, tumor

    Below RR can indicate: Chronic viral or bacterial infection, active infection, oxidative stress, suppressed bone marrow production or post bone marrow transplant while recovering, hepatitis

Eosinophils (% and 10^3/uL) are a type of white blood cell. Eosinophil count can help monitor mistletoe therapy; eosinophil count should rise slightly approximately six weeks into mistletoe therapy.

    RR: 0–7% of total WBC

    Above RR can indicate: Intestinal parasites, food or environmental allergy, asthma. This measurement can also be elevated with graft-versus-host disease or post bone marrow transplant

    Below RR can indicate: Stress

Monocytes (% and 10^3/uL) are a type of white blood cell that remove dead or damaged cells and help fight cancer cells.

    RR: <7%

Basophils (% and 10^3/uL) are a type of white blood cell that help your body defend against allergens.

    RR: 0–1%

The Neutrophil to Lymphocyte Ratio (NLR) is a general indication of immune function. In healthy people, it is about (2:1). A lower neutrophil to lymphocyte ratio is associated with blood cancers. A higher neutrophil to lymphocyte ratio can be a negative prognostic factor in many cancers and is also associated with adverse overall survival in solid tumors.[1] Monitoring this ratio during cancer treatment offers an indication of whether the immune system is becoming overstressed by treatment. It is also valuable to monitor the NLR postconventional treatment.

To arrive at this ratio, divide the absolute neutrophil count (not the percentage) by the absolute lymphocyte count (again, not the percentage). Be sure you are using the absolute count and not the percentage, as the CBC includes both.

Platelets

Blood Platelet Count (10^3/uL) measures the number of platelets in the blood. Platelets are small, colorless cell fragments necessary for clotting.

Reference range (RR): 155–385 10^3/uL

Above RR can indicate: Dehydration, chronic leukemia or malignancy, arthritis, acute infections, types of anemia, oral contraceptives, blood loss, iron deficiency, stress response

Below RR can indicate: Infections, immune thrombocytopenia (ITP), heavy metal burden, a response to certain drugs, leukemia, liver dysfunction, circadian rhythm dysfunction

Comprehensive Metabolic Panel (CMP)

The CMP is a blood test that offers a snapshot of the body's chemistry. It typically includes the following measurements:

Albumin (g/dL) is one of the major blood proteins produced in the liver. A low albumin is highly linked to a poor prognosis in many cancers. If your child's albumin drops below 3 you should also inquire about an IV albumin infusion for your child while you work on identifying the root cause of their low albumin and healing the cause. Studies show that pretreatment of lower albumin is a predictor of lower survival; this alone is a huge argument for preparing for treatment and not rushing in. Take the time to raise your child's albumin before anticancer therapy starts. Serum albumin is a predictor of bone marrow transplant course pretransplant and of overall survival post-transplant.[2]

Reference range (RR): 4–5.5 g/dL

Above RR can indicate: Dehydration

Below RR can indicate: Hypochlorhydria, liver dysfunction, oxidative
stress, vitamin C deficiency, protein deficiency

Alkaline Phosphatase (U/L) (ALP) is a group of isoenzymes that originate
in the bone, liver, skin, and placenta. If there is a significant elevation in this
marker, it should be followed up by testing ALP isoenzymes, which will help
pinpoint the tissue involved.

RR: 105–420 U/L, but dependent on age

Above RR may indicate: Biliary obstruction, liver cell damage, bone loss
or increased bone turnover, rheumatoid arthritis, Hodgkin lymphoma, bone growth, leaky gut, shingles, metastatic carcinoma of the
bone, vitamin C deficiency

Below RR may indicate: Zinc deficiency, drug causes (especially certain
medications that block estrogen), hypothyroidism

Alanine Aminotransferase (U/L) (ALT) is an enzyme present in high concentrations in the liver and, to a lesser extent, skeletal muscle, the heart, and
the kidneys.

RR: 10–30 U/L

Above RR may indicate: Liver dysfunction, cirrhosis of the liver, liver cell
damage, liver damage from chemotherapy/immunotherapy, biliary
tract obstruction, excessive muscle breakdown, aspirin poisoning,
metastatic carcinoma, pancreatitis

Below RR may indicate: Vitamin B6 deficiency, fatty liver, liver congestion, protein deficiency, malabsorption

Anion Gap (mEq/L) measures the gap (or difference) between negatively
and positively charged electrolytes in the blood. It is used to get a sense of
tissue acidity or alkalinity.

RR: 7–12 mEq/L

Above RR may indicate: Acidosis, which can be from dehydration,
kidney disease, ketoacidosis

Below RR may indicate: Low albumin, certain cancers, kidney problem,
liver disease, heart disease

Aspartate Aminotransferase (AST) (U/L) is an enzyme present in highly
metabolic tissues like the liver, heart, kidney, and lungs.

RR: 10–30 U/L

Above RR may indicate: Developing congestive heart failure, liver cell
damage, liver dysfunction, excessive muscle breakdown, viral infection
such as Epstein-Barr virus or cytomegalovirus (CMV), metastatic cancer, pancreatitis, damage to liver from chemotherapy/immunotherapy

Above RR may indicate: Vitamin B6 deficiency, protein deficiency,
malabsorption, kidney failure

Blood Urea Nitrogen (BUN) (mg/dL) reflects kidney function. The BUN/
creatinine ratio is a further indicator of kidney function.

RR: 10–16 mg/dL

Above RR can indicate: Renal disease, renal insufficiency

Below RR can indicate: Dehydration, hypochlorhydria, adrenal hyperfunction, dysbiosis, edema, drug reaction (especially diuretics and
steroids), anterior pituitary dysfunction, low-protein diet, malabsorption, pancreatic insufficiency, liver dysfunction

Carbon Dioxide (mEq/L) is a measure of bicarbonate in the blood.

RR: 25–30 mEq/L

Above RR can indicate: Metabolic acidosis, adrenal hyperfunction,
hypochlorhydria, respiratory acidosis, fever, vomiting, diuretics drugs

Below RR can indicate: Metabolic acidosis, vitamin B1 deficiency, respiratory alkalosis, dehydration, diabetes

Chloride (mEq/L) is an electrolyte, used as a general measure of tissue
acidity or alkalinity.

RR: 100–106 mEq/L

Above RR can indicate: Metabolic acidosis, adrenal hyperfunction,
dehydration

Below RR can indicate: Hypochlorhydria, metabolic alkalosis, adrenal
hypofunction, drug causes (steroids, laxatives, and diuretics)

Creatinine (mg/dL) reflects kidney function. Creatinine is important because
many chemotherapy drugs, as well as imaging contrast, are cleared by the
kidneys. It's important to keep your child well hydrated and pay attention
not only to the normal value of the lab, but the baseline value for your child.

RR: <1.1, but dependent on age

Above RR can indicate: Urinary tract congestion or obstruction, renal
disease, renal insufficiency, UTI, drug reactions

Below RR can indicate: Liver disease, muscle atrophy, malnutrition, cachexia

Glucose (mg/dL) measures blood sugar. When glucose is at or above 100 mg/dL, a hemoglobin A1c (HgA1c) test, which measures average blood sugar over approximately 120 days, should be ordered.

RR: 55–90 mg/dL

Above RR can indicate: Prediabetes, diabetes, insulin resistance, stress, fatty liver, drug reaction, especially steroids

Below RR can indicate: Hypoglycemia related to liver issues, hyperinsulinism, adrenal hypofunction

Potassium (mEq/L) is an indicator of, among other things, adrenal hormone function.

RR: 4–4.5 mEq/L

Above RR can indicate: Adrenal hypofunction, dehydration, tissue destruction, metabolic acidosis, respiratory distress

Below RR can indicate: Adrenal hyperfunction, diuretic drugs response, hypertension

Serum Calcium (mg/dL) measures calcium in the body. The majority of calcium is stored in bones and teeth, but the body does also maintain calcium in the blood.

RR: 9.2–10.0 mg/dL

Above RR can indicate: Parathyroid hyperfunction, thyroid hypofunction, impaired cell membrane death, neoplasm, vitamin D3 excess or vitamin D3 excess without enough vitamin K2

Below RR can indicate: Parathyroid hypofunction, calcium need, hypochlorhydria, vitamin D3 insufficiency, osteoporosis

Serum Phosphorus (mg/dL) measures the amount of phosphate in the blood. The majority of phosphorus in the body is stored with calcium in the bone.

RR: 3–4 mg/dL

Above RR can indicate: Parathyroid hypofunction, bone growth or bone repair, diet excessive in phosphate, renal insufficiency

Below RR can indicate: Parathyroid hyperfunction, hypochlorhydria, hyperinsulinism, diet high in carbohydrates

Sodium (mEq/L) can be affected by changes in fluid balance.

RR: 135–142 mEq/L

Above RR can indicate: Adrenal hyperfunction, Cushing disease,
  dehydration, drug causes (steroids, NSAIDS, laxatives, antihypertensives)
Below RR can indicate: Adrenal hypofunction, Addison's disease, edema,
  drug diuretics, drug causes (heparin, laxatives, diuretics)

Total Bilirubin (mg/dL) can indicate excessive red blood cell destruction or liver dysfunction. Direct conjugated and indirect unconjugated bilirubin should be checked if total bilirubin is elevated. When direct is elevated, this indicates that the biliary tract or liver is involved, and when indirect is elevated this is from RBC hemolysis.

RR: <1.1 as per scale (depends on your child's age)
Above RR can indicate: Biliary stasis, oxidative stress, liver dysfunction,
  RBC hemolysis, Gilbert's syndrome, heavy metal burden
Below RR can indicate: Prolonged fasting

Total Globulin (g/dL) can be used to investigate digestive disturbances and/or inflammatory disturbances.

RR: 2.4–2.8 g/dL
Above RR can indicate: Hypochlorhydria, liver dysfunction, oxidative
  stress, heavy metal toxicity, immune activation, parasites
Below RR can indicate: Digestive dysfunction or inflammation,
  immune insufficiency

Total Protein (g/dL) can be an indication of nutritional deficiencies, digestive disorders, and dehydration. Children going through cancer treatment often do not get enough protein in their diet and become malnourished. Additionally, treatment causes malabsorption. Without healing the gut, children will have an ongoing struggle to absorb the protein they are eating. Focus on feeding your child high-quality protein and healing the gut. This is very important during and after treatment.

RR: 6.9–7.4 g/dL
Above RR can indicate: Dehydration, diabetes
Below RR can indicate: Hypochlorhydria, digestive dysfunction and
  inflammation, liver dysfunction, diet low in protein, malabsorption

Trifecta Labs

As I covered in chapter 3, there are three conventional lab tests, known as the "trifecta labs," that offer tremendous insight into the efficacy of treatment and progress toward healing. Dr. Nasha Winters is credited for pioneering the use of these three labs together to assess and tweak integrative treatment protocols. I have repeated summary information here about each lab, as well as reference ranges, and more specifics on LDH isoenzymes.

C-Reactive Protein (CRP) is a protein found in the plasma whose concentrations increase when there is inflammation in the body. If elevated, CRP can indicate multiple drug resistance or side effects from the treatment. CRP is very important and should be used through standard-of-care treatment and beyond.

Reference range (RR): <1

Above RR may indicate: Inflammation, infection, cancer

Erythrocyte Sedimentation Rate (ESR) is useful for determining level of tissue destruction. This test shows us how sticky our blood is. Elevated ESR is common in autoimmune disease.

RR: 0–15 mm/hour

Above RR can indicate: Tissue inflammation or destruction,
    arthritis, cardiovascular conditions, active allergy, mononucleosis,
    malignant disease

Lactate Dehydrogenase (LDH) is an enzyme of the anaerobic metabolic pathway. When it increases, it can indicate tissue damage. It also suggests if the body's terrain is "welcoming" to cancer, and it is a tumor marker for lymphoma and leukemia. For solid tumors it helps us evaluate the tumor microenvironment and tells us the rate of cell division. It can also indicate damage to organs such as the liver, lungs, heart, or kidneys. For more specifics, ask your child's metabolic oncology practitioner to order an LDH isoenzyme (see below).

Do note, however, that LDH can often be elevated in kids when they are going through a growth spurt. This would typically show as elevated isoenzymes LDH 1 and LDH 2. For this reason, LDH is less reliable as an inflammatory marker for children than it is for adults.

RR: 140–200 U/L (or as per scale)

Above RR may indicate: Liver/biliary obstruction, cardiovascular
    disease, vitamin B12 deficiency, anemia, tissue inflammation, tissue
    destruction, viral infection, malignant neoplasm, spreading cancer

Below RR may indicate: Reactive hypoglycemia, excess vitamin C

LDH Isoenzymes

LDH 1: Heart, red blood cells
RR: 10–34%

LDH 2: Heart, lymph, red blood cells
RR: 30–45%

LDH 3: Pulmonary, spleen, adrenals, kidney, pancreas
RR: 13–27%

LDH 4: Hepatic, skeletal muscle, skin
RR: 2–14%

LDH 5: Hepatic, skeletal muscle, skin
RR: 6–15%
Elevated LDH 1, 2, and 3, and a decrease in LDH 5 may indicate leukemia.

Serum Ferritin

Serum ferritin, the protein that stores iron in your blood, is the body's main iron storage site. Many pediatric cancer patients end up with iron overload from blood transfusions. The initial treatment for this is therapeutic phlebotomy—weekly bloodletting—to decrease the serum ferritin. If serum ferritin is over 1,000 nanograms per milliliter, an MRI should be ordered to assess iron deposits in organs such as the liver and heart. If serum ferritin is high, your metabolic oncology practitioner should investigate the cause with a Total Serum Iron test and Total Iron Binding Capacity test (TIBC) to evaluate for cause of low ferritin.

Reference range (RR): 35–75 mcg/dL

Above RR may indicate: Hemochromatosis (iron overload), excess consumption of iron, inflammation/liver dysfunction, blood transfusions, vitamin B12 deficiency, hemolytic anemia

Below RR may indicate: Iron deficiency/anemia

Homocysteine

High homocysteine levels can be due to genetic or epigenetic factors, such as the MTHRF SNP, vitamin B12, B6, and folate deficiencies, or hypothyroidism. Testing is inexpensive and may prompt your child's metabolic oncology practitioner to test for epigenetics mutation of MTHFR and support accordingly.

Reference range (RR): 5–7 umol/L

Above RR may indicate: Vitamin deficiency, malabsorption, leaky gut, MTHFR SNP, drug reaction, renal dysfunction, malignant neoplasm, psoriasis, osteoporosis

Below RR may indicate: Malnutrition, malabsorption, vitamin B deficiency, poor production of glutathione

Thyroid

Thyroid-Stimulating Hormone (TSH) is used to evaluate thyroid function.

Reference range (RR): 0.35–2.5 uU/ml

Above RR may indicate: Hypothyroidism, medications causes, autoimmune thyroid disease, pituitary tumor

Below RR may indicate: Hyperthyroidism, heavy metal burden, drug side effects (including to steroids), Graves' disease, Hashimoto's thyroiditis

Total T3 measures the level of triiodothyronine (T3) in the blood. T3 is the active thyroid hormone, produced from the conversion of thyroxine (T4) in the peripheral tissue.

RR: 60–230 ng/dL

Above RR may indicate: Hyperthyroidism, iodine deficiency, protein malnutrition, liver or renal disease

Below RR may indicate: Primary hypothyroidism, selenium deficiency, liver disease, drug or radiation therapy for hyperthyroidism

Total T4 measures the level of thyroxine, or T4, a hormone secreted by the thyroid gland.

RR: 6–12 mcg/dL

Above RR may indicate: Hyperthyroidism, thyroid replacement, drug causes

Below RR may indicate: Primary hypothyroidism, iodine deficiency, reaction to steroids, drug causes

Vitamin D3

The 25-hydroxy vitamin D blood test measures the amount of vitamin D3 in the blood.

Reference range (RR): 50–100 IU

Above RR may indicate: Oversupplementation

Below RR may indicate: Undersupplementation, malabsorption

Serum Magnesium

To get an accurate magnesium level you should check RBC magnesium.

Reference range (RR): 1.6–2.5 mg/dL

Above RR can indicate: Renal dysfunction, thyroid hypofunction, dehydration

Below RR can indicate: Epilepsy, muscle spasm, liver dysfunction, malabsorption, inflammation, post bone marrow transplant sign of kidneys needing more recovery time

Hemoglobin A1c (HgA1c)

This test measures average blood sugar over approximately 120 days.

Reference range (RR): 4.8–5.2%

Above RR can indicate: Diabetes or prediabetes, lead toxicity

Below RR can indicate: Hypoglycemia

Gamma-Glutamyl Transpeptidase (GGTP)

GGTP is an enzyme that is present in various organs, including the kidneys, pancreas, spleen, heart, and brain, but is present in the highest amounts in the liver.

Reference range (RR): 10–30 U/L

Above RR may indicate: Dysfunction inside of the liver and biliary dysfunction, liver cell damage, alcohol damage, pancreatitis, pancreatic insufficiency, parasites, diabetes, liver metastases, veno-occlusive disease, liver damage

Below RR may indicate: Vitamin B6 deficiency, magnesium need, protein deficiency, malabsorption

Epigenetic Testing

At the time of this writing, Nutrition Genome offers an epigenetic test for $359. This is the test that I use the most in my practice, as it offers one hundred clinically relevant genes for whole-body analysis. It is easy and relatively inexpensive for a lot of useful information, including information on SNPs like MTHFR and PON1 (see chapter 3). This test is often the basis of many of my recommendations for individual nutritional needs and supplements. It is not necessary to order this test through your child's integrative oncology practitioner; however, the practitioner should be very helpful in interpreting the results and developing recommendations based on them.

The test itself consists of a simple cheek swab delivered to your home, and turnaround time is about three to five weeks. If possible, it is best to conduct this test before chemotherapy or radiation begins, but it can also be done after treatment has started.

Brand: Nutrition Genome
Website: https://nutritiongenome.com
Test name: DNA Test Kit & Health Report

Microbiome Tests

There are a number of companies that offer microbiome/gut health test kits. I recommend these four.

Brand: Mosaic Diagnostics
Test name: OAT (Organic Acid Test)
Type: Urine
Turnaround time: 3–4 weeks
Cost: Approximately $100
Ordered by practitioner: Yes
Offers: Metabolic snapshot of patient's overall health, including markers for vitamin and mineral levels, as well as intestinal yeast and bacteria; snapshot of gut health

Brand: Diagnostic Solutions Laboratory
Test name: Organic Acid Test (OAT)
Type: Stool
Turnaround time: 3–4 weeks
Cost: Approximately $300
Ordered by practitioner: Yes
Offers: Detection of parasites, bacteria, and fungi by targeting the specific DNA of the organisms tested

Brand: Genova Diagnostics
Test name: GI Effects
Type: Stool
Turnaround time: 3–4 weeks
Cost: Depends on insurance
Ordered by practitioner: Yes

Offers: A visual and colorful snapshot identifying maldigestion, inflammation, dysbiosis, metabolite imbalance, and infection

Brand: Diagnostic Solutions Laboratory
Test name: GI-Map
Type: Stool
Turnaround time: 4–6 weeks
Cost: Depends on insurance
Ordered by practitioner: Yes
Offers: Good and bad bacteria in stool, parasites

Food Sensitivity Tests

If an elimination diet doesn't provide the needed answers, I sometimes order food sensitivity testing through the following company:

Brand: Cyrex Laboratories
Test name: Cyrex Array 10
Type: Blood
Turnaround time: 4–6 weeks
Cost: $300–$800
Ordered by practitioner: Yes
Offers: Many options for food sensitivity testing

Toxicity Tests

Brand: MosaicDX
Test name: Glyphosate
Type: Urine
Turnaround time: 4–6 weeks
Cost: Approximately $100
Ordered by practitioner: Yes
Information it gives: Glyphosate exposure

Brand: MosaicDX
Test name: Toxic Nonmetal Chemicals
Type: Urine
Turnaround time: 4–6 weeks
Cost: Approximately $500

Ordered by practitioner: Yes
Offers: Screens for 173 different environmental pollutants using eighteen
   different metabolites

Heavy Metal Tests

Brand: MosaicDX
Test name: Metals Urine Test
Type: Urine
Turnaround time: 4–6 weeks
Cost: Approximately $100
Ordered by practitioner: Yes
Offers: Levels of common heavy metals

Hormone Testing

Brand: DUTCH Test
Test name: Dutch Complete
Type: Urine
Turnaround time: 4–6 weeks
Cost: Approximately $400
Ordered by practitioner: Yes
Offers: Levels of estrogen, progesterone, and testosterone, adrenal
   hormones, melatonin, and more

Immune System Testing

Brand: Cyrex Laboratories
Test name: The Lymphocyte Map
Type: Blood draw
Turnaround time: 4–6 weeks.
Cost: Approximately $400
Ordered by practitioner: Yes
Offers: A broad picture of the immune status

Sample Recipes and Meal Plans

MEAL PLANNING CAN BE OVERWHELMING FOR ANY FAMILY EVEN WHEN cancer is not a factor. In my experience, nutrition is often the most stressful part of implementing changes. I have found having the right tools in our kitchen is key. Invest in a good quality blender like a Vitamix. Buy a stainless-steel slow cooker and an electronic pill crusher. Write out a list of your child's favorite foods for every meal and then seek out recipes that make these in a healthier way. You may be looking for a grain-free version, such as paleo or keto pancakes. In this way, you are still providing your child their favorite foods but with healthier ingredients.

I have found that if you involve your child in making food, they are more likely to eat it. There are many nutritious "keto" desserts you can make together and enjoy. I cannot stress enough the value of preparing food as a family. Fun plates and music and chef hats go a long way.

Sample Grocery List

Vegetables

Avocados	Cucumbers	Onions
Asparagus	Eggplant	Parsley
Bok choy	Garlic	Radishes
Broccoli	Green beans	Snow peas
Brussels sprouts	Jalapeños	Spinach
Cabbage	Kale	Zucchini
Cauliflower	Lettuce	
Celery	Mushrooms	

Fats

Almond butter	Coconut cream	Macadamia oil
Almond oil	Coconut milk	Mayonnaise
Avocado oil	Flaxseed oil	MCT oil
Butter	Hemp seed oil	Olive oil
Coconut oil	Macadamia butter	Peanut butter

Nuts/Seeds

Almond milk	Coconut	Pecans
Almonds	Flaxseed	Pepitas
Brazil nuts	Hemp seeds	Sunflower seeds
Chia seeds	Macadamias	Walnuts

Dairy and Eggs

Full-fat Greek yogurt	sheep, or goats	Sour cream
Full-fat organic raw	Heavy cream	
milk from cows,	Organic, soy-free eggs	

Cheese

Blue cheese	Cream cheese	Mozzarella
Cheddar	Feta	Parmesan
Cottage cheese	Goat cheese	Ricotta

Meat

Beef	Lamb	Turkey
Bison	Organ meats	
Chicken	Pork	

Seafood

Anchovies	Sardines	Wild salmon
Crab	Shrimp	
Lobster	Tuna	

Fruit

Blueberries	Peaches	Strawberries
Cantaloupe	Raspberries	Watermelon

Recipes

Each of these recipes makes one serving, and they are made the same way:
Combine all the ingredients in a blender and blend until smooth.

Easy Breezy Super Soup (feeding tube only)

2 cups homemade bone broth

½ avocado, sliced

1 tablespoon MCT oil, or olive oil if coconut allergy

1 scoop high-quality collagen powder

1 serving beef liver capsules, removed from capsules

Easy Breezy Super Soup Variation (feeding tube only)

2 cups homemade bone broth

4 ounces chicken liver, beef liver, duck liver, or wild salmon, chopped

2 stalks asparagus, chopped, or ¼ cup chopped organic seasonal vegetables

1 bunch parsley or cilantro, leaves only

2 to 3 tablespoons ghee, MCT oil, or olive oil

½ cup full-fat kefir (optional)

Anti-Cachexia Formula

10 to 60 grams MCT oil

1 to 5 grams omega-3 oil

1 serving mixed amino acid powder

1 gram carnitine

1 gram turmeric

1 serving B-complex vitamins

IV vitamin-mineral formula with amino acid infusion

Anti-Cachexia Smoothie

2 cups filtered water with ice, herbal tea, or homemade almond milk

2 tablespoons high-quality collagen powder

1 tablespoon ground flax seeds

1 tablespoon MCT oil

¼ to ½ avocado, sliced

2 tablespoons protein powder, such as PaleoProtein

1 teaspoon vanilla

1 teaspoon omega-3 oil

1 teaspoon amino acid powder

Sample Menus

Below you'll find some sample menus. As a reminder, Foundation Nutrition is a healthy diet—it's what we should all be eating, cancer or not. Level 1 Nutrition removes grains, refined sugar, and legumes and can be used to transition into and out of ketosis. Level 2 Nutrition puts you into ketosis and should be done with the guidance of an experienced practitioner. Foundation Nutrition and Level 1 Nutrition plans are easier to follow and allow for more diversity. I have provided a meal plan for Level 2 Nutrition both without a feeding tube and with a feeding tube. There is no feeding tube sample menu for Foundation Nutrition or Level 1 Nutrition because most kids that have a feeding tube are at a place where they're likely following Level 2 Nutrition already.

Foundation Nutrition

Breakfast	Organic, soy-free chicken or duck eggs with organic turkey sausage	Organic, soaked-spelt pancakes with whipped cream and seasonal berries	Blend full-fat organic yogurt and protein powder into a shake with frozen mango slices and 1 tsp MCT oil
Lunch	Homemade tomato soup with Parmesan cheese crackers	Cheese quesadilla made with an organic, sprouted tortilla and home-made guacamole	Homemade mac and cheese with organic 100% millet noodles and cheddar cheese, sauerkraut on the side
Dinner	Grass-fed steak with steamed broccoli topped with butter, side of sprouted organic black rice	Homemade bone broth with buckwheat ramen, organic chicken, cooked carrot, broccoli, and green onion	Tacos made from sprouted tortillas with grass-fed ground beef and cabbage, home-made guacamole

Snack	Celery sticks with homemade almond butter	Organic carrot sticks, sliced cucumbers, and bell pepper strips with homemade ranch dressing	Organic olives, green or black

Level 1 Nutrition

Breakfast	Organic, soy-free chicken or duck eggs with organic turkey sausage	Almond flour pancakes with keto-friendly syrup	Full-fat organic kefir with wild blueberries, MCT oil, protein powder, and monk fruit
Lunch	Cheese quesadilla made with an almond-flour tortilla and organic full-fat cheese, guacamole, side of fermented carrots	Homemade bone broth broccoli-cheese soup thickened with tapioca	Wrap with nitrate-free organic ham and cheese, mustard, in an almond flour tortilla, side of sauerkraut
Dinner	Organic 100% millet pasta with pesto and side salad with fermented beets	Grain-free hard taco shells with grass-fed ground beef and lettuce, tomatoes, sauerkraut	Baked wild salmon, baked sweet potato with butter, side of fermented beets
Snack	Berries with homemade whipped heavy cream	Almond crackers with sliced cheese and olives	Baked organic apple with cinnamon

Level 2 Nutrition (without feeding tube)

Breakfast	Organic soy-free eggs with 1 slice nitrate-free bacon	Almond flour pancakes with keto-friendly syrup	Low-carb, high-protein waffle with whipped cream and berries
Lunch	Low-carb wrap with chicken and veggies	Organic, nitrate-free hot dog (no bun), with mustard and sauerkraut	Bone broth soup with keto-friendly noodles and veggies
Dinner	Stir-fry with veggies, ghee, and cauliflower rice	Grass-finished burgers (no bun)	Salad with home-made bone-broth veggie soup
Snack	Keto-friendly popsicle	A scoop of Mammoth Creameries ice cream	Lily's dark chocolate or SuperFat cookies

Level 2 Nutrition (with feeding tube)

Breakfast	½ to 1 Functional Formularies Keto Sustain pouch thinned with quality water or home-made bone broth	1 cup homemade bone broth blended with ½ avocado and protein powder	1 cup bone broth with 1 tablespoon MCT oil and 2 scoops collagen protein powder
Lunch	4 to 8 ounces Super Soup	4 to 8 ounces Super Soup	Serenity Kids bison pouch thinned with homemade bone broth or quality water
Dinner	½ to 1 Functional Formularies Keto Peptide	1 pouch Functional Formularies Keto Peptide	1 pouch Functional Formularies Keto Peptide
Snack	¼ cup berries with sugar-free whipped cream	Green olives	Keto crackers with cheese slices

Sample Inpatient Packing Lists for Patients and Caregivers

You have stopped, breathed, and made essential decisions about the approach you would like to take for your child's treatment. You have conducted the appropriate testing. Now it is time to prepare your family for treatment. Most children with cancer will spend some time in the hospital. That could be days, weeks, or months, depending on your child's treatment plan. Preparation is key in order to minimize stress and drawbacks and maximize the benefits. Here are some recommendations for what to bring.

Patient Packing List

- Comfortable nontoxic pajamas. They should be 100 percent cotton and never treated with flame retardant. There are special pajamas made for ports and PICC lines.
- Comfortable nontoxic clothing. It is important, especially with longer stays, to maintain healthy routines as much as possible. Your child should get dressed in the morning.
- A cotton pillowcase
- Electronics, such as an iPad or laptop with wired headphones and EMF protection. Always keep a blanket between the device and your child's lap.
- A soft-bristled toothbrush and organic toothpaste
- Organic toiletries, including shampoo, body wash, and body butter
- Slippers and walking shoes
- Crafts/journal/Legos: something other than electronics that your child enjoys
- Ball to play catch or balloons to toss around and get your child moving
- Heat pack
- Castor oil pack
- Nutrient-dense snacks, including keto-friendly popsicles for post-chemo mouth sores
- Small rebounder (trampoline)
- Organic tube-feeding formula (if applicable); see appendix B for recommendations

Caregiver Packing List

- Organic coffee, tea, and/or herbal beverages
- Air filter
- Pill crusher and cutter
- Supplements (organized)
- Notepad for keeping track of supplements for each day and other data
- Folders to organize your child's medical plan and labs; I prefer clear ones
- Journal/devotional/book
- Headphones, so you can listen to audiobooks, podcasts, music, and meditations
- Nutrient-dense snacks
- Small blender, such as a Magic Bullet, for smoothies, tube feeding, or pills that require blending
- Water filter or bottles of filtered water
- Yoga mat and walking shoes
- Organic toiletries, including shampoo, body wash, and body butter for both parent and child
- Your own cotton pillow, sheets, and blankets
- Frozen nutrient-dense dinners and treats that you can keep in a shared freezer
- Cutting board
- Utensils
- Soup bowl and paper plates
- Hot plate, air fryer, and mini refrigerator if your facility does not have a kitchen

I recommend that you ask friends or family members to bring you the following items every day: bone broth, fresh organic nutrient-dense meals, a big hug, and, once in a while, a break to run home, do something for yourself, and hold your other people.

Recommended Resources

Find a Metabolic Oncology Practitioner

Believe Big

www.believebig.org

www.believebig.org/integrative-practitioner

Founded by Ivelisse Page, a stage 4 colon cancer survivor, wife, and mother of four, Believe Big's mission is to "bridge the gap between conventional and complementary medicine for fighting cancer."

Metabolic Terrain Institute of Health

www.mtih.org

www.terrain.network

Founded by Dr. Nasha Winters, Steve Ottersberg, and Cindy Kennedy, the Metabolic Terrain Institute of Health's mission is to "ingrain the terrain-based treatment methodology into cancer treatment and preventative care through practice, science, research, education, training, collaboration and funding."

Zuza's Way Integrative Care

www.zuzasway.com

This is my integrative health practice. On the website, you will find my favorite resources and information on online consultancy or becoming a patient.

Websites and Organizations

Kick Cancer

www.kickcancermovement.org

www.seasonjohnson.com

Founded by Season Johnson, a functional nutritional therapy practitioner and mom of a cancer survivor, Kick Cancer "educates and empowers families on nutrition and natural wellness to complement during and after cancer treatment." Johnson is a recipient of the Weston A. Price Foundation Activist Award and the Nutritional Therapy Association's Children's Health Advocate Award for her work with pediatric cancer. Her focus is on real food, supplementation, detoxification, and cleaning up the environment. Her website offers a wealth of information including a podcast, meal planning, and consultancy.

The MaxLove Project
www.maxloveproject.org
The Max Love Project is "dedicated to improving the quality of life of families facing childhood cancers, pediatric rare diseases, and chronic hospitalizations with evidence-based culinary medicine, integrative care, and emotional health."

The Stern Method
www.thesternmethod.com
Ryan and Teddy Sternagel developed the Stern Method after their one-year-old son, Ryder, was diagnosed with stage 4 neuroblastoma. The method includes "super nutrition, targeted supplementation, energy medicine and healthy lifestyle practices," along with the building of an "anti-cancer home."

Diet and Nutrition

The Charlie Foundation for Ketogenic Therapies
https://charliefoundation.org
"The Charlie Foundation for Ketogenic Therapies was founded in 1994 to provide information about diet therapies for people with epilepsy, other neurological disorders and select cancers."

Dietary Therapies
www.dietarytherapies.com
Dietary Therapies offers "nutritional strategies for cancer and metabolic health."

Remission Nutrition
www.remissionnutrition.com
Remission Nutrition has been "consulting on the forefront of metabolic oncology nutrition therapy since 2010."

Weston A. Price Foundation
www.westonaprice.org
"The Weston A. Price Foundation (WAPF) is your source for accurate information on nutrition and health, always aiming to provide the scientific validation of traditional foodways."

Food and Supplement Suppliers

Azure Standard
www.azurestandard.com
Azure Standard is "a natural health food distributor bringing bulk and specialty health foods to communities all across the nation."

A Campaign for Real Milk
www.realmilk.com
"A Campaign for Real Milk was founded by raw milk activists in 1998 and launched as a website in 1999. The Weston A. Price Foundation adopted A Campaign for Real Milk as a project in January 2000."

Eat Wild
www.eatwild.com
Eat Wild was founded by Jo Robinson in 2001 "to promote the many advantages of raising livestock on pasture on small family farms. . . . It is now the #1 clearinghouse in the United States for science-based information about pasture-based farming. The site features a state-by-state (plus Canada) directory of local farmers who meet Eat Wild's criteria."

FarmMatch
www.farmmatch.com
Farm Match is a resource to find small farms and buying clubs near you.

Ketone IQ
https://hvmn.com

LocalHarvest
www.localharvest.org
"Local Harvest connects people looking for good food with the farmers who produce it."

The Seasonal Food Guide
www.seasonalfoodguide.org
The Seasonal Food Guide is "designed to help you find out what produce is in season in your state throughout the year."

Thrive Market
www.thrivemarket.com
Thrive Market is a US e-commerce membership-based retailer offering natural and organic food products.

Full-Spectrum Hemp Products and CBD Oil

Twisted River Farms
www.twistedriverfarms.com
Twisted River Farms is my family's online shop for our organically grown hemp and CBD products.

EMF Safety

Alpha Labs Trifield EMF Meter Model TF2
www.trifield.com/product/trifield-emf-meter

OMPERIO Smart Meter Cover
https://omperio.com/smart-meter-cover

EMF Academy
http://emfacademy.com

The Stern Method: Household EMF Sources and Solutions
www.thesternmethod.com/household-emf-sources-and-solutions-cell-phone-radiation-wi-fi-electric-fields-smart-meters

Probiotics

Ther-Biotic Complete Probiotic from Klaire Labs
Ther-Biotic Kid's Chewable from Klaire Labs
Vital-10 Probiotic from Klaire Labs
Ortho Biotic from Ortho Molecular Products
Probiotic G.I. from Pure Encapsulations
MetaKids Probiotic from Metagenics

Probiotic Synergy from Designs for Health
Probiotic Pearls from Integrative Therapeutics
FloraPro-LP Probiotic from Thorne

Books

*The Metabolic Approach to Cancer: Integrating Deep Nutrition, the Ketogenic Diet,
and Nontoxic Bio-Individualized Therapies* by Dr. Nasha Winters and Jess
Higgins Kelley

Conversations with God by Neale Walsch

*The End to Upside Down Thinking: Dispelling the Myth That the Brain Produces
Consciousness, and the Implications for Everyday Life* by Mark Gober

Living Untethered: Beyond the Human Predicament by Michael A. Singer

Mistletoe and the Emerging Future of Integrative Oncology by Dr. Steven Johnson
and Dr. Nasha Winters

*Outside the Box Cancer Therapies: Alternative Therapies That Treat and Prevent
Cancer* by Dr. Paul Anderson and Dr. Mark Stengler

Naturopathic Oncology: An Encyclopedic Guide for Patients and Physicians by Dr.
Neil McKinney

The Vaccine Book: Making the Right Decision for Your Child by Dr. Robert
W. Sears

Vaccines, Autoimmunity, and the Changing Nature of Childhood Illness by
Dr. Thomas Cowan

*The Vaccine-Friendly Plan: Dr. Paul's Safe and Effective Approach to Immunity and
Health from Pregnancy through Your Child's Teen Years* by Dr. Paul Thomas
and Jennifer Margulis

What's in the Way Is the Way: A Practical Guide for Waking Up to Life by
Mary O'Malley

Financial and Material Support

Mitchell Thorp Foundation
www.mitchellthorp.org
The Mitchell Thorpe Foundation is dedicated to "supporting families whose
children suffer from life-threatening illnesses, diseases, and disorders by providing financial, emotional and resource support to their desperate situation."

The Cancer Response Team

www.cancerresponseteam.org

"Cancer Response Team, Inc. is . . . dedicated to helping children get supportive cancer care. [They] do so by providing their families with financial assistance for integrative and complementary cancer therapies from time of diagnosis up to six months post treatment."

Carsyn Neille Foundation

www.carsynneillefoundation.org

The Carsyn Neille Foundation "design[s] sustainable, nontoxic bedrooms that improve the quality of life and thrivorship of families."

Alex's Lemonade Stand

www.alexslemonade.org

The Alex's Lemonade Stand foundation's mission is "to change the lives of children with cancer through funding impactful research, raising awareness, supporting families and empowering everyone to help cure childhood cancer."

Warrior Wagons

www.warriorwagonsinc.com

Warrior Wagons' "mission is simple yet powerful: to provide newly diagnosed pediatric cancer families with a collapsible wagon filled with practical and comfort items to help them on their cancer journey."

Bridges of Gold

www.bridgesofgold.com

"Through voice, partnerships and accessibility [Bridges of Gold is] working to empower and build the childhood cancer community."

Special Spaces

www.specialspaces.org

Special Spaces "create[s] dream bedroom makeovers for dependent children ages 2–19 with cancer who are within one year of treatment."

Retreats and Camps

Starlite Shores Family Camp

www.starliteshores.org

Starlite Shores Family Camp's mission is "to serve families living through childhood cancer with the love of Christ, offering them an environment to be relaxed, be renewed, and be restored as a family."

Lighthouse Family Retreat
www.lighthousefamilyretreat.org
Lighthouse Family Retreat is "a faith-based non-profit that exists to strengthen every family living through childhood cancer. [They] host restorative retreats and develop helpful resources so that families and their support systems can find hope in God and help in their fight."

Meditation and Spirituality

Sarah Blondin
www.sarahblondin.com

Sez Kristiansen
www.sezkristiansen.com

Notes

Chapter 1. Stop and Breathe

1. "What Is Cancer?," National Cancer Institute, May 5, 2021, https://www.cancer.gov/about-cancer/understanding/what-is-cancer.
2. Douglas Hanahan, "Hallmarks of Cancer: New Dimensions," *Cancer Discovery* 12, no. 1 (2022): 31–46, https://doi.org/10.1158/2159-8290.cd-21-1059.
3. Carlos Sonnenschein and Ana M. Soto, "Somatic Mutation Theory of Carcinogenesis: Why It Should Be Dropped and Replaced," *Molecular Carcinogenesis* 29, no. 4 (2001): 205–11, https://doi.org/10.1002/1098-2744(200012)29:4<205::aid-mc1002>3.0.co;2-w.
4. Angela M. Otto, "Warburg Effect(s)—A Biographical Sketch of Otto Warburg and His Impacts on Tumor Metabolism," *Cancer & Metabolism* 4, no. 1 (2016), https://doi.org/10.1186/s40170-016-0145-9.
5. Thomas N. Seyfried, "Cancer as a Mitochondrial Metabolic Disease," *Frontiers in Cell and Developmental Biology* 3 (2015), https://doi.org/10.3389/fcell.2015.00043.
6. Andrew M. Seaman, "Life-Extending Capacity of New Cancer Drugs Varies Widely," *Reuters*, January 2, 2017, https://www.reuters.com/article/us-health-cancer-drugs/life-extending-capacity-of-new-cancer-drugs-varies-widely-idUSKBN14M16G.
7. Sebastian Salas-Vega, Othon Iliopoulos, and Elias Mossialos, "Assessment of Overall Survival, Quality of Life, and Safety Benefits Associated with New Cancer Medicines," *JAMA Oncology* 3, no. 3 (2017): 382–90, https://doi.org/10.1001/jamaoncol.2016.4166.

Chapter 2. Build Out the Team

1. You can order an epigenetic test called the DNA Test Kit & Whole Body Health Report from the Nutrition Genome website (https://nutritiongenome.com/shop-nutrition-ge-nome/ref/973). A kit will be mailed to your home, where you can perform a cheek swab on your child and send it back. In a few weeks you will get very valuable information on your child's epigenetics that can help you make better decisions for your child's treatment and treatment doses and support.
2. Christina Signorelli et al., "Childhood Cancer Survivors' Reported Late Effects, Motivations for Seeking Survivorship Care, and Patterns of Attendance," *Oncologist* 28, no. 5 (2023): 276–86, https://doi.org/10.1093/oncolo/oyad004.
3. Thomas P. Ahern et al., "Medication-Associated Phthalate Exposure and Childhood Cancer Incidence, *Journal of the National Cancer Institute* 114, no. 6 (2022): 885–94, https://doi.org/10.1093/jnci/djac045; Mei Chen et al., "Residential Exposure to Pesticide During Childhood and Childhood Cancers: A Meta-Analysis," *Pediatrics* 136, no. 4 (2015): 719–29, https://doi.org/10.1542/peds.2015-0006; Margeaux Epner et al., "Understanding the Link between Sugar and Cancer: An Examination of the Preclinical and Clinical Evidence," *Cancers* 14, no. 24 (2022): 6042, https://doi.org/10.3390/cancers14246042.

4. Kumar Ganesan, Kumeshini Sukalingam, and Baojun Xu, "Impact of Consumption of Repeatedly Heated Cooking Oils on the Incidence of Various Cancers—A Critical Review," *Critical Reviews in Food Science and Nutrition* 59, no. 3 (2017): 488–505, https://doi.org/10.1080/10408398.2017.1379470.

Chapter 3. Conduct Additional Testing

1. Michael F. Holick, "Vitamin D and Sunlight: Strategies for Cancer Prevention and Other Health Benefits," *Clinical Journal of the American Society of Nephrology* 3, no. 5 (2008): 1548–54, https://doi.org/10.2215/cjn.01350308; Michell Fullmer et al., "Newly Diagnosed Children with Cancer Have Lower 25-Vitamin D Levels than Their Cancer-Free Peers: A Comparison across Age, Race, and Sex," *Cancers* 14, no. 10 (2022): 2378, https://doi.org/10.3390/cancers 14102378; Heidi Godman, "Vitamin D Supplements May Reduce Risk of Invasive Cancer," *Harvard Health*, June 1, 2021, https://www.health.harvard.edu/cancer/vitamin-d-supplements -may-reduce-risk-of-invasive-cancer; Hun Ju Lee et al., "Low 25(OH) Vitamin D₃ Levels Are Associated with Adverse Outcome in Newly Diagnosed, Intensively Treated Adult Acute Myeloid Leukemia," *Cancer* 120, no. 4 (2013): 521–29, https://doi.org/10.1002/cncr.28368.

2. Mariarosaria Negri et al., "Vitamin D-Induced Molecular Mechanisms to Potentiate Cancer Therapy and to Reverse Drug-Resistance in Cancer Cells," *Nutrients* 12, no. 6 (2020): 1798, https://doi.org/10.3390/nu12061798; Natalja Jackmann et al., "Vitamin D Status in Children with Leukemia," *Blood* 132 (Supplement 1) (2018): 3973, https://doi.org /10.1182/blood-2018-99-119557.

3. Bing Zhu and Shen Qu, "The Relationship Between Diabetes Mellitus and Cancers and Its Underlying Mechanisms," *Frontiers in Endocrinology* 13 (2022), https://www.ncbi.nlm. nih.gov/pmc/articles/PMC8873103; Centers for Disease Control and Prevention, "New Research Uncovers Concerning Increases in Youth Living with Diabetes in the U.S.," CDC (press release), August 24, 2021, https://archive.cdc.gov/#/details?url=https:// www.cdc.gov/media/releases/2021/p0824-youth-diabetes.html.

4. Monica Jimenez, "Only 7% of American Adults Have Good Cardiometabolic Health," *Tufts Now*, July 5, 2022, https://now.tufts.edu/2022/07/05/only-7-american-adults-have -good-cardiometabolic-health.

5. Mohamed Badr et al, "Insulin-like Growth Factor-1 and Childhood Cancer Risk," *Oncology Letters* 1, no. 6 (2010): 1055–60, https://doi.org/10.3892/ol.2010.169.

6. Netanya I. Pollock and Laurie E. Cohen, "Growth Hormone Deficiency and Treatment in Childhood Cancer Survivors," *Frontiers in Endocrinology* 12 (2021), https://doi .org/10.3389/fendo.2021.745932.

7. Atsushi Makimoto et al., "Magnesium Supplementation Therapy to Prevent Cisplatin-Induced Acute Nephrotoxicity in Pediatric Cancer: A Protocol for a Randomized Phase 2 Trial," *Contemporary Clinical Trials Communications* 16 (2019): 100440, https://doi .org/10.1016/j.conctc.2019.100440.

8. Rosaura Gutiérrez-Vargas et al., "Effect of Zinc on Oropharyngeal Mucositis in Children with Acute Leukemia Undergoing Chemotherapy," *Medicina Oral Patología Oral Y Cirugia Bucal* 25, no. 6 (2020): e791–98, https://doi.org/10.4317/medoral.23798.

9. Vinit C. Shanbhag et al., "Copper Metabolism as a Unique Vulnerability in Cancer," *Biochimica et Biophysica Acta (BBA)—Molecular Cell Research* 1868, no. 2 (2021): 118893, https://doi.org/10.1016/j.bbamcr.2020.118893; Gutiérrez-Vargas, "Effect of Zinc."

10. Edwin A. Takahashi et al., "Nephrotoxicity of Gadolinium-Based Contrast in the Setting of Renal Artery Intervention: Retrospective Analysis with 10-Year Follow-Up," *Diagnostic and Interventional Radiology* 24, no. 6 (2018): 378–84, https://doi.org/10.5152/dir.2018.18172.

11. Moshe Rogosnitzky and Stacy Branch, "Gadolinium-Based Contrast Agent Toxicity: A Review of Known and Proposed Mechanisms," *BioMetals* 29, no. 3 (2016): 365–76, https://doi.org/10.1007/s10534-016-9931-7.

12. Institute for Functional Medicine, "IFM's Elimination Diet: Personalized Optimized Nutrition," https://www.ifm.org/news-insights/heal-the-gut-with-the-ifm-elimination-diet.

13. Karin Ried, Peter Eng, and Avni Sali, "Screening for Circulating Tumour Cells Allows Early Detection of Cancer and Monitoring of Treatment Effectiveness: An Observational Study," *Asian Pacific Journal of Cancer Prevention* 18, no. 8 (2017): 2275–85, https://doi.org/10.22034/APJCP.2017.18.8.2275.

Chapter 4. Assess the Terrain

1. Nasha Winters and Jess Higgins Kelley, *The Metabolic Approach to Cancer: Integrating Deep Nutrition, the Ketogenic Diet, and Nontoxic Bio-Individualized Therapies* (White River Junction, VT: Chelsea Green, 2017).

2. Christina Gillezeau et al., "The Evidence of Human Exposure to Glyphosate: A Review," *Environmental Health* 18, no. 1 (2019): 2, https://doi.org/10.1186/s12940-018-0435-5.

3. Gillezeau et al., "The Evidence of Human Exposure to Glyphosate."

4. Maria A. Karalexi et al., "Exposure to Pesticides and Childhood Leukemia Risk: A Systematic Review and Meta-Analysis," *Environmental Pollution* 285 (2021): 117376, https://doi.org/10.1016/j.envpol.2021.117376.

5. Karalexi et al., "Exposure to Pesticides and Childhood Leukemia Risk."

6. Deven M. Patel et al., "Residential Proximity to Agriculture and Risk of Childhood Leukemia and Central Nervous System Tumors in the Danish National Birth Cohort," *Environment International* 143 (2020): 105955, https://doi.org/10.1016/j.envint.2020.105955.

7. Andrew Nguyen, "Residential Proximity to Plant Nurseries and Risk of Childhood Leukemia," *Environmental Research* 200 (2021): 111388, https://doi.org/10.1016/j.envres.2021.111388.

8. Jackson Holtz, "UW Study: Exposure to Chemical in Roundup Increases Risk for Cancer," *UW News*, February 13, 2019, https://www.washington.edu/news/2019/02/13/uw-study-exposure-to-chemical-in-roundup-increases-risk-for-cancer.

9. Preetha Anand et al., "Cancer Is a Preventable Disease That Requires Major Lifestyle Changes" *Pharmaceutical Research* 25 (2008):2097–2116, http://doi.org/10.1007/s11095-008-9661-9.

Chapter 5. Address the Terrain

1. "Family Cancer Syndromes," American Cancer Society, September 14, 2022, https://www.cancer.org/healthy/cancer-causes/genetics/family-cancer-syndromes.html.

2. Ming Zhao et al., "MTHFR Gene Polymorphisms and Methotrexate Toxicity in Adult Patients with Hematological Malignancies: A Meta-Analysis," *Pharmacogenomics* 17, no. 9 (2016): 1005–17, https://doi.org/10.2217/pgs-2016-0004.

3. Dave Levitan, "Three SNPs Associated with Overall Survival in Pediatric Ewing Sarcoma," *Cancer Network,* June 24, 2016, https://www.cancernetwork.com/view/three-snps -associated-overall-survival-pediatric-ewing-sarcoma.

4. Angela Gutierrez-Camino et al., "Involvement of SNPs in miR-3117 and miR-3689d2 in Childhood Acute Lymphoblastic Leukemia Risk," *Oncotarget* 9, no. 33 (2018): 22907–14, https://doi.org/10.18632/oncotarget.25144.

5. Salma A. Bargal et al., "Genome-Wide Association Analysis Identifies SNPs Predictive of *in Vitro* Leukemic Cell Sensitivity to Cytarabine in Pediatric AML," *Oncotarget* 9, no. 79 (2018): 34859–75, https://doi.org/10.18632/oncotarget.26163.

6. Matthew Eng, "Is This Detox Gene Protecting You from Pesticides? (PON1)" *Selfdecode,* September 9, 2019, https://selfdecode.com/app/article/detox-pesticides-pon1.

7. Edward Giovannucci et al., "Diabetes and Cancer: A Consensus Report," *Diabetes Care* 33, no. 7 (2010): 1674–85, https://doi.org/10.2337/dc10-0666.

8. American Heart Association, "How Much Sugar Is Too Much?," Heart Attack and Stroke Symptoms, accessed September 14, 2022, https://www.heart.org/en/healthy-living /healthy-eating/eat-smart/sugar/how-much-sugar-is-too-much.

9. Giovannucci, "Diabetes and Cancer."

10. Centers for Disease Control and Prevention, "1 in 5 Adolescents and 1 in 4 Young Adults Now Living with Prediabetes," CDC (press release), December 2019, https://archive.cdc .gov/#/details?url=https://www.cdc.gov/media/releases/2019/p1202-diabetes.html.

11. Claudio Vernieri et al., "Fasting-Mimicking Diet plus Chemotherapy in Breast Cancer Treat-ment," *Nature Communications* 11, no. 1 (2020), https://doi.org/10.1038/s41467-020-18194-1.

12. Sara Goodman, "Tests Find More Than 200 Chemicals in Newborn Umbilical Cord Blood," *Scientific American,* December 2, 2009, https://www.scientificamerican.com /article/newborn-babies-chemicals-exposure-bpa.

13. Jennifer 8. Lee, "Some Carcinogens Are Seen as Greater Risk to Children," *New York Times,* March 4, 2003, https://www.nytimes.com/2003/03/04/us/some-carcinogens -are-seen-as-greater-risk-to-children.html.

14. Sandee LaMotte, "Sunscreen Recall: What the Finding of a Cancer-Causing Chemical Means for You," *CNN Health,* July 17, 2021, https://www.cnn.com/2021/07/17/health /sunscreen-recall-cancer-wellness.

15. Tara Strand, "Johnson & Johnson," *Mesothelioma.com,* accessed September 14, 2022, https://www.mesothelioma.com/asbestos-exposure/companies/johnson-and-johnson.

16. Carly Hyland et al., "Organic Diet Intervention Significantly Reduces Urinary Pesticide Levels in U.S. Children and Adults," *Environmental Research* 171 (2019): 568–75, https://doi.org/10.1016/j.envres.2019.01.024.

17. Catherine Saint Louis, "Scrutiny for Laxatives as a Childhood Remedy," *New York Times,* Janu-ary 5, 2015, https://www.nytimes.com/2015/01/06/science/scrutiny-for-a-childhood-remedy. html; Roland B. Walter et al., "Long-Term Use of Acetaminophen, Aspirin, and Other Nonsteroidal Anti-Inflammatory Drugs and Risk of Hematologic Malignancies: Results from the Prospective Vitamins and Lifestyle (VITAL) Study," *Journal of Clinical Oncology* 29, no. 17 (2011): 2424–31, https://doi.org/10.1200/jco.2011.34.6346; Arnaldo C. Couto et al., "Pregnancy, Maternal Exposure to Analgesic Medicines, and Leukemia in Brazilian Children Below 2 Years of Age," *European Journal of Cancer Prevention* 24, no. 3 (2015): 245–52, https:// doi.org/10.1097/CEJ.0000000000000070; "Long-Term Anti-Inflammatory Drug Use May

Increase Cancer-Related Deaths for Certain Patients," *ScienceDaily*, December 19, 2016, https://www.sciencedaily.com/releases/2016/12/161219134400.htm.

18. Anahad O'Connor, "New York Attorney General Targets Supplements at Major Retailers," *New York Times*, February 3, 2015, https://archive.nytimes.com/well.blogs.nytimes.com/2015/02/03/new-york-attorney-general-targets-supplements-at-major-retailers.

19. Robert Snyder, "Leukemia and Benzene," *International Journal of Environmental Research and Public Health* 9, no. 8 (2012): 2875–93, https://doi.org/10.3390/ijerph9082875.

20. Sharon Ruth Skolnick, "Exposing Airports' Poison Circles," *Earth Island Journal*, 2000–2001, https://www.us-caw.org/pdf/expair.pdf.

21. Anne Brice, "Moskowitz: Cellphone Radiation Is Harmful, but Few Want to Believe It," *Berkeley News*, July 1, 2021, https://news.berkeley.edu/2021/07/01/health-risks-of-cell-phone-radiation.

22. Aadra P. Bhatt, Matthew R. Redinbo, and Scott J. Bultman, "The Role of the Microbiome in Cancer Development and Therapy," *CA: A Cancer Journal for Clinicians* 67, no. 4 (2017): 326–44, https://doi.org/10.3322/caac.21398.

23. Ewen Callaway, "C-Section Babies Are Missing Key Microbes," *Nature*, September 18, 2019, https://doi.org/10.1038/d41586-019-02807-x.

24. Sasha Milbeck, "C-Section Birth Associated with Numerous Health Conditions," *National Center for Health Research*, December 7, 2020, https://www.center4research.org/c-section-birth-health-risks.

25. Mayo Clinic, "Mayo Clinic: Antibiotics Before Age 2 Associated with Chronic Childhood Health Problems," *SciTechDaily*, November 15, 2020, https://scitechdaily.com/mayo-clinic-antibiotics-before-age-2-associated-with-chronic-childhood-health-problems.

26. Aneta Sevcikova et al., "The Impact of the Microbiome on Resistance to Cancer Treatment with Chemotherapeutic Agents and Immunotherapy," *International Journal of Molecular Sciences* 23, no. 1 (2022): 488, https://doi.org/10.3390/ijms23010488.

27. Romain Daillère et al., "*Enterococcus hirae* and *Barnesiella intestinihominis* Facilitate Cyclophosphamide-Induced Therapeutic Immunomodulatory Effects," *Immunity* 45, no. 4 (2016): 931–43, https://doi.org/10.1016/j.immuni.2016.09.009.

28. "Valisure Detects Benzene in Hand Sanitizers," Valisure, March 24, 2021, https://www.valisure.com/valisure-newsroom/valisure-detects-benzene-in-hand-sanitizers.

29. Arhanti Sadanand, Jason G. Newland, and Jeffrey J. Bednarski, "Safety of Probiotics Among High-Risk Pediatric Hematopoietic Stem Cell Transplant Recipients," *Infectious Diseases and Therapy* 8, no. 2 (2019): 301–6, https://doi.org/10.1007/s40121-019-0244-3.

30. Giuseppe L. Banna et al., "*Lactobacillus rhamnosus* GG: An Overview to Explore the Rationale of Its Use in Cancer," *Frontiers in Pharmacology* 8 (2017), https://doi.org/10.3389/fphar.2017.00603.

31. Shanley Pierce, "Does Acetaminophen Cause Cancer?" *TMC News*, May 6, 2020, https://www.tmc.edu/news/2020/05/does-acetaminophen-cause-cancer.

32. Yoshikazu Kinoshita, Norihisa Ishimura, and Shunji Ishihara, "Advantages and Disadvantages of Long-Term Proton Pump Inhibitor Use," *Journal of Neurogastroenterology and Motility* 24, no. 2 (2018): 182–96, https://doi.org/10.5056/jnm18001.

33. Luke Mountjoy et al., "Proton Pump Inhibitors Associated with Higher Incidence of Mucositis in Patients Receiving Methotrexate for Graft vs Host Disease Prophylaxis," *Blood* 134 (Supplement 1) (2019): 3262. https://doi.org/10.1182/blood-2019-128644.

34. Winters and Kelley, *The Metabolic Approach to Cancer*, 171.
35. Daniel Ruiz and Heather Patisaul, eds., "Endocrine Disrupting Chemicals (EDCs)," Endocrine Society, last updated January 24, 2022, https://www.endocrine.org/patient-engagement/endocrine-library/edcs.
36. Erika Edwards, "Anxiety, Depression Rampant Among Children Even Before the Pandemic," *NBC News*, February 24, 2022, https://www.nbcnews.com/health/health-news/anxiety-depression-rampant-children-even-pandemic-rcna17545; Sarah Molano, "Youth Depression and Anxiety Doubled During the Pandemic, New Analysis Finds," *CNN Health*, August 10, 2021, https://www.cnn.com/2021/08/10/health/covid-child-teen-depression-anxiety-wellness; Nicole Racine et al., "Global Prevalence of Depressive and Anxiety Symptoms in Children and Adolescents During COVID-19: A Meta-Analysis," *JAMA Pediatrics* 175, no. 11 (2021): 1142–50, https://doi.org/10.1001/jamapediatrics.2021.2482.
37. "Suicide," National Institute of Mental Health, 2021, https://www.nimh.nih.gov/health/statistics/suicide.
38. Shirui Dai et al., "Chronic Stress Promotes Cancer Development," *Frontiers in Oncology* 10 (2020), https://doi.org/10.3389/fonc.2020.01492.
39. Myrthala Moreno-Smith, Susan K. Lutgendorf, and Anil K. Sood, "Impact of Stress on Cancer Metastasis," *Future Oncology* 6, no. 12 (2010): 1863–81, https://doi.org/10.2217/fon.10.142.

Chapter 6. Develop a Nutrition Plan

1. "Dirty Dozen: EWG's 2023 Shopper's Guide to Pesticides in Produce," Environmental Working Group, 2023, https://www.ewg.org/foodnews/dirty-dozen.php.
2. Catherine Roberts, "An Easy Way to Remove Pesticides," *Consumer Reports*, October 25, 2017, https://www.consumerreports.org/pesticides-herbicides/easy-way-to-remove-pesticides-a3616455263.
3. "What Chemicals Are Lurking in Your Loaf? Nearly Two Thirds of Bread Products Found to Contain Pesticide Residues," *DailyMail*, July 17, 2014, https://www.dailymail.co.uk/news/article-2695224/What-chemicals-lurking-loaf-Nearly-two-thirds-bread-products-contain-pesticide-residues.html.
4. Alexis Tempkin and Olga Naidenko, "Glyphosate Contamination in Food Goes Far Beyond Oat Products," Environmental Working Group, February 28, 2019, https://www.ewg.org/news-insights/news/glyphosate-contamination-food-goes-far-beyond-oat-products.
5. Tempkin and Naidenko, "Glyphosate Contamination."
6. Chensheng Lu et al., "Organic Diets Significantly Lower Children's Dietary Exposure to Organophosphorus Pesticides," *Environmental Health Perspectives* 114, no. 2 (2005): 260–63, https://doi.org/10.1289/ehp.8418.
7. "Study Associates Organic Food Intake in Childhood with Better Cognitive Development," *Neuroscience News*, June 30, 2021, https://neurosciencenews.com/child-cognition-organic-diet-18840.
8. US Department of Agriculture, "Dietary Guidelines for Americans 2020–2025," https://www.dietaryguidelines.gov/sites/default/files/2020-12/Dietary_Guidelines_for_Americans_2020-2025.pdf.

9. Hongqiang Wang et al., "[Research Progress of the Inhibitory Effect of Deuterium-Depleted Water on Cancers]," *Nan Fang Yi Ke Da Xue Xue Bao [Journal of Southern Medical University]* 32, no. 10 (2012), https://pubmed.ncbi.nlm.nih.gov/23076183.

10. Kehinde Adekola, Steven T. Rosen, and Mala Shanmugam, "Glucose Transporters in Cancer Metabolism," *Current Opinion in Oncology* 24, no. 6 (2012): 650–54, https://doi.org/10.1097/CCO.0b013e328356da72; Maria V. Liberti and Jason W. Locasale, "The Warburg Effect: How Does It Benefit Cancer Cells?," *Trends in Biochemical Sciences* 41, no. 3 (2016): 211–18, https://doi.org/10.1016/j.tibs.2015.12.001; Quangdon Tran et al., "Revisiting the Warburg Effect: Diet-Based Strategies for Cancer Prevention," *BioMed Research International* 2020, https://doi.org/10.1155/2020/8105735.

11. Sidra Naveed, Muhammad Aslam, and Aftab Ahmad, "Starvation Based Differential Chemotherapy: A Novel Approach for Cancer Treatment," *Oman Medical Journal* 29, no. 6 (2014): 391–98, https://doi.org/10.5001/omj.2014.107.

12. Rainer Johannes Klement, "Fasting, Fats, and Physics: Combining Ketogenic and Radiation Therapy against Cancer," *Complementary Medicine Research* 25, no. 2 (2018): 102–13, https://doi.org/10.1159/000484045. Ketogenic diet protecting healthy cells against chemotherapy: Wamidh Talib et al., "Ketogenic Diet in Cancer Prevention and Therapy: Molecular Targets and Therapeutic Opportunities," *Current Issues in Molecular Biology* 43, no. 2 (2021): 558–89, https://doi.org/10.3390/cimb43020042. Ketogenic diet can prolong survival time in cancer: Jing Li, Haiyan Zhang, and Zhu Dai, "Cancer Treatment with the Ketogenic Diet: A Systematic Review and Meta-Analysis of Animal Studies," *Frontiers in Nutrition* 8 (2021), https://www.frontiersin.org/articles/10.3389/fnut.2021.594408/full. Ketogenic diet and reduced drug toxicity: Francesco Plotti et al., "Diet and Chemotherapy: The Effects of Fasting and Ketogenic Diet on Cancer Treatment," *Chemotherapy* 65, no. 3–4 (2020): 77–84, https://doi.org/10.1159/000510839. Ketogenic diet and better quality of life: Melanie Schmidt et al., "Effects of a Ketogenic Diet on the Quality of Life in 16 Patients with Advanced Cancer: A Pilot Trial," *Nutrition and Metabolism* 8 (2011), https://doi.org/10.1186/1743-7075-8-54.

13. Anastasia Dressler et al., "The Ketogenic Diet Including Breast Milk for Treatment of Infants with Severe Childhood Epilepsy: Feasibility, Safety, and Effectiveness," *Breastfeeding Medicine* 15, no. 2 (2020): 72–78, https://doi.org/10.1089/bfm.2019.0190.

14. Simone Dal Bello et al., "Ketogenic Diet in the Treatment of Gliomas and Glioblastomas," *Nutrients* 14, no. 18 (2022): 3851, https://doi.org/10.3390/nu14183851; Kenneth A. Schwartz et al., "Long Term Survivals in Aggressive Primary Brain Malignancies Treated with an Adjuvant Ketogenic Diet," *Frontiers in Nutrition* 9 (2022), https://www.frontiersin.org/articles/10.3389/fnut.2022.770796; Karisa C. Schreck et al., "Feasibility and Biological Activity of a Ketogenic/Intermittent-Fasting Diet in Patients with Glioma," *Neurology* 97, no. 9 (2021): e953–63, https://doi.org/10.1212/WNL.0000000000012386.

15. Stefanie de Groot et al., "Effects of Short-Term Fasting on Cancer Treatment," *Journal of Experimental & Clinical Cancer Research* 38, no. 1 (2019), https://doi.org/10.1186/s13046-019-1189-9; Daniela Koppold-Liebscher et al., "Short-Term Fasting Accompanying Chemotherapy as a Supportive Therapy in Gynecological Cancer: Protocol for a Multicenter Randomized Controlled Clinical Trial," *Trials* 21, no. 1 (2020), https://doi.org/10.1186/s13063-020-04700-9.

16. Jana Wells et al., "Efficacy and Safety of a Ketogenic Diet in Children and Adolescents with Refractory Epilepsy—A Review," *Nutrients* 12, no. 6 (2020): 1809, https://doi.org/10.3390/nu12061809; Se Hee Kim et al., "The Ketogenic Diet in Children 3 Years of Age or Younger: A 10-Year Single-Center Experience," *Scientific Reports* 9, no. 1 (2019): 8736, https://doi.org/10.1038/s41598-019-45147-6.

17. Schmidt et al., "Effects of a Ketogenic Diet"; Alexandre Perez et al., "Ketogenic Diet Treatment in Diffuse Intrinsic Pontine Glioma in Children: Retrospective Analysis of Feasibility, Safety, and Survival Data," *Cancer Reports* 4, no. 5 (2021): e1383, https://doi.org/10.1002/cnr2.1383.

18. Masahiro Maeyama et al., "Metabolic Changes and Anti-Tumor Effects of a Ketogenic Diet Combined with Anti-Angiogenic Therapy in a Glioblastoma Mouse Model," *Scientific Reports* 11, no. 1 (2021), https://doi.org/10.1038/s41598-020-79465-x; Daniela D. Weber et al., "Ketogenic Diet in the Treatment of Cancer—Where Do We Stand?" *Molecular Metabolism* 33 (2020) : 102–21, https://doi.org/10.1016/j.molmet.2019.06.026.

19. Jana Wells et al., "Efficacy and Safety of a Ketogenic Diet."

Chapter 7. Evaluate General Integrative Therapies

1. Zoë Slote Morris, Steven Wooding, and Jonathan Grant, "The Answer Is 17 Years, What Is the Question: Understanding Time Lags in Translational Research," *Journal of the Royal Society of Medicine* 104, no. 12 (2011): 510–20, https://doi.org/10.1258/jrsm.2011.110180.

2. Lavinia Fiorentino and Sonia Ancoli-Israel, "Sleep Dysfunction in Patients with Cancer," *Current Treatment Options in Neurology* 9, no. 5 (2010): 337–46, https://www.ncbi.nlm.nih.gov/pmc/articles/PMC2951736.

3. Lindsay M. H. Steur, "Sleep-Wake Rhythm Disruption Is Associated with Cancer-Related Fatigue in Pediatric Acute Lymphoblastic Leukemia," *Sleep* 43, no. 6 (2019), https://doi.org/10.1093/sleep/zsz320.

4. Valerie F. Gladwell, "The Great Outdoors: How a Green Exercise Environment Can Benefit All," *Extreme Physiology & Medicine* 2, no. 1 (2013), https://doi.org/10.1186/2046-7648-2-3; Caoimhe Twohig-Bennett and Andy Jones, "The Health Benefits of the Great Outdoors: A Systematic Review and Meta-Analysis of Greenspace Exposure and Health Outcomes," *Environmental Research* 166 (2018): 628–37, https://doi.org/10.1016/j.envres.2018.06.030.

5. Qing Li, "Effect of Forest Bathing Trips on Human Immune Function," *Environmental Health and Preventive Medicine* 15, no. 1 (2009): 9–17, https://doi.org/10.1007/s12199-008-0068-3.

6. Ye Wen et al., "Medical Empirical Research on Forest Bathing (*Shinrin-yoku*): A Systematic Review," *Environmental Health and Preventative Medicine* 24 (2019), https://doi.org/10.1186/s12199-019-0822-8.

7. James Oschman, Gaetan Chevalier, and Richard Brown, "The Effects of Grounding (Earthing) on Inflammation, the Immune Response, Wound Healing, and Prevention and Treatment of Chronic Inflammatory and Autoimmune Diseases," *Journal of Inflammation Research* (2015): 83–96, https://doi.org/10.2147/jir.s69656.

8. Javier S. Morales et al., "Inhospital Exercise Training in Children with Cancer: Does It Work for All?," *Frontiers in Pediatrics* 6 (2018): 404, https://doi.org/10.3389/fped.2018.00404.

9. Erika Mora et al., "Vincristine-Induced Peripheral Neuropathy in Pediatric Cancer Patients," *American Journal of Cancer Research* 6, no. 11 (2016): 2416–30, https://www.ncbi.nlm.nih.gov/pmc/articles/PMC5126263.

10. Mora et al., "Vincristine-Induced Peripheral Neuropathy."

11. Debra Reis and Tisha Throne Jones, "Frankincense Essential Oil as a Supportive Therapy for Cancer-Related Fatigue: A Case Study," *Holistic Nursing Practice* 32, no. 3 (2018): 140–42, https://doi.org/10.1097/hnp.0000000000000261.

12. Byoungduck Park et al., "Boswellic Acid Suppresses Growth and Metastasis of Human Pancreatic Tumors in an Orthotopic Nude Mouse Model through Modulation of Multiple Targets," *PLoS ONE* 6, no. 10 (2012): e26943, https://doi.org/10.1371/journal.pone.0026943.

13. Tamara T. Lah, "Cannabigerol Is a Potential Therapeutic Agent in a Novel Combined Therapy for Glioblastoma," *Cells* 10, no. 2 (2021): 340, https://doi.org/10.3390/cells10020340; Gerard Nahler, "Cannabidiol and Other Phytocannabinoids as Cancer Therapeutics," *Pharmaceutical Medicine* 36 (2022): 99–129, https://doi.org/10.1007/s40290-022-00420-4.

14. James M. Nichols and Barbara L. F. Kaplan, "Immune Responses Regulated by Cannabidiol," *Cannabis and Cannabinoid Research* 5, no. 1 (2020), https://doi.org/10.1089/can.2018.0073.

15. Linda A. Parker, Erin M. Rock, and Cheryl L. Limebeer, "Regulation of Nausea and Vomiting by Cannabinoids," *British Journal of Pharmacology* 163, no. 7 (2010): 1411–22, https://doi.org/10.1111/j.1476-5381.2010.01176.x.

16. Kimberly A. Babson, James Sottile, and Danielle Morabito, "Cannabis, Cannabinoids, and Sleep: A Review of the Literature," *Current Psychiatry Reports* 19, no. 23 (2017), https://doi.org/10.1007/s11920-017-0775-9.

17. Howard Meng et al., "Cannabis and Cannabinoids in Cancer Pain Management," *Current Opinion in Supportive & Palliative Care* 14, no. 2 (2020): 87–93, https://doi.org/10.1097/spc.0000000000000493.

18. Sarah Walker and Samantha Velez, "Can Marijuana Potentially Improve Inflammation Symptoms?" Veriheal, accessed September 16, 2022, https://www.veriheal.com/conditions/inflammation.

19. Moshe Yeshurun et al., "Cannabidiol for the Prevention of Graft-Versus-Host-Disease after Allogeneic Hematopoietic Cell Transplantation: Results of a Phase II Study," *Biology of Blood and Marrow Transplantation* 21, no. 10 (2015): 1770–75, https://doi.org/10.1016/j.bbmt.2015.05.018.

20. Sayeda Yasmin-Karim et al., "Enhancing the Therapeutic Efficacy of Cancer Treatment with Cannabinoids," *Frontiers in Oncology* 8 (2018): 114, https://doi.org/10.3389/fonc.2018.00114.

21. Yasmin-Karim et al., "Enhancing the Therapeutic Efficacy."

22. Anitra C. Carr and Silvia Maggini, "Vitamin C and Immune Function," *Nutrients* 9, no. 11 (2017): 1211, https://www.ncbi.nlm.nih.gov/pmc/articles/PMC5707683.

23. Fullmer, "Newly Diagnosed Children with Cancer."

24. Orsolya Juhász et al., "Examining the Vitamin D Status of Children with Solid Tumors," *Journal of the American College of Nutrition* 39, no. 2 (2019): 128–34, https://doi.org/10.1080/07315724.2019.1616233.

25. Miklós Garami et al., "Fermented Wheat Germ Extract Reduces Chemotherapy-Induced Febrile Neutropenia in Pediatric Cancer Patients," *Journal of Pediatric Hematology/Oncology* 26, no. 10 (2004): 631–35, https://pubmed.ncbi.nlm.nih.gov/15454833.

26. Tracey Yeend et al., "The Effectiveness of Fermented Wheat Germ Extract as an Adjunct Therapy in the Treatment of Cancer: A Systematic Review," *JBI Library of Systematic Reviews* 10, no. 42 (2012): 1–12, https://doi.org/10.11124/jbisrir-2012-289.

27. Bonny Burns-Whitmore et al., "Alpha-Linolenic and Linoleic Fatty Acids in the Vegan Diet: Do They Require Dietary Reference Intake/Adequate Intake Special Consideration?" *Nutrients* 11, no. 10 (2019): 2365, https://doi.org/10.3390/nu11102365; Katie E. Lane et al., "Bioavailability and Conversion of Plant Based Sources of Omega-3 Fatty Acids—A Scoping Review to Update Supplementation Options for Vegetarians and Vegans," *Critical Reviews in Food Science and Nutrition* 62, no. 18 (2021): 4982–97, https://doi.org/10.1080/10408398.2021.1880364.

28. Raquel D. S. Freitas and Maria M. Campos, "Protective Effects of Omega-3 Fatty Acids in Cancer-Related Complications," *Nutrients* 11, no. 5 (2019): 945, https://doi.org/10.3390/nu11050945; Saraswoti Khadge, "Immune Regulation and Anti-Cancer Activity by Lipid Inflammatory Mediators," *International Immunopharmocology* 65 (2018): 580–92, https://doi.org/10.1016/j.intimp.2018.10.026; Jahnabi Roy et al., "Antitumorigenic Properties of Omega-3 Endocannabinoid Epoxides," *Journal of Medicinal Chemistry* 61, no. 13 (2018): 5569–79, https://doi.org/10.1021/acs.jmedchem.8b00243.

29. Alexandra Podpeskar et al., "Omega-3 Fatty Acids and Their Role in Pediatric Cancer," *Nutrients* 13, no. 6 (2021): 1800, https://doi.org/10.3390/nu13061800.

30. Freitas and Campos, "Protective Effects of Omega-3 Fatty Acids"; Khadge, "Immune Regulation and Anti-Cancer"; Roy et al., "Antitumorigenic Properties of Omega-3 Endocannabinoid Epoxides."

31. Podpeskar et al., "Omega-3 Fatty Acids and Their Role."

32. Peter M. Anderson and Rajesh V. Lalla, "Glutamine for Amelioration of Radiation and Chemotherapy Associated Mucositis during Cancer Therapy," *Nutrients* 12, no. 6 (2020): 1675, https://doi.org/10.3390/nu12061675.

33. E. Ward et al., "Oral Glutamine in Paediatric Oncology Patients: A Dose Finding Study," *European Journal of Clinical Nutrition* 57, no. 1 (2003): 31–36, https://doi.org/10.1038/sj.ejcn.1601517.

34. Yasushi Honda et al., "Efficacy of Glutathione for the Treatment of Nonalcoholic Fatty Liver Disease: An Open-Label, Single-Arm, Multicenter, Pilot Study," *BMC Gastroenterology* 17 (2017), https://doi.org/10.1186/s12876-017-0652-3.

35. Alexis D. Leal et al., "North Central Cancer Treatment Group/Alliance Trial N08CA—The Use of Glutathione for Prevention of Paclitaxel/Carboplatin-Induced Peripheral Neuropathy: A Phase 3 Randomized, Double-Blind, Placebo-Controlled Study," *Cancer* 120, no. 12 (2014): 1890–97, https://doi.org/10.1002/cncr.28654.

36. "Helleborus Therapy," *Helixor*, March 2022, https://helixor.com/helleborus-therapy.

37. Linda Elsegood, ed., *The LDN Book: How a Little-Known Generic Drug—Low Dose Naltrexone—Could Revolutionize Treatment for Autoimmune Diseases, Cancer, Autism, Depression, and More* (White River Junction, VT: Chelsea Green Publishing, 2016).

38. "What Is LDN?," LDN Research Trust, accessed September 16, 2022, https://ldnresearchtrust.org.

39. "Low Dose Naltrexone (LDN) Therapy," Medicor Cancer Centres, October 21, 2019, https://medicorcancer.com/ldn-therapy.

40. "Low Dose Naltrexone (LDN) Therapy Can Help Treat Patients with Cancer," American Integrative Pharmacy, January 9, 2022, https://www.americanintegrative.com/low-dose-naltrexone-ldn-therapy-can-help-treat-patients-with-cancer.

41. Wamidh H. Talib et al., "Melatonin in Cancer Treatment: Current Knowledge and Future Opportunities," *Molecules* 26, no. 9 (2021): 2506, https://doi.org/10.3390/molecules26092506.

42. Jie Deng et al., "N-Acetylcysteine Decreases Malignant Characteristics of Glioblastoma Cells by Inhibiting Notch2 Signaling," *Journal of Experimental & Clinical Research* 38, no. 2 (2019), https://doi.org/10.1186/s13046-018-1016-8.

43. Seema Patel and Arun Goyal, "Recent Developments in Mushrooms as Anti-Cancer Therapeutics: A Review," *3 Biotech* 2, no. 1 (2012): 1–15, https://doi.org/10.1007/s13205-011-0036-2.

44. İnayet Güntürk et al., "The Effect of N-Acetylcysteine on Inflammation and Oxidative Stress in Cisplatin-Induced Nephrotoxicity: A Rat Model," *Turkish Journal of Medical Sciences* 49, no. 6 (2019), https://doi.org/10.3906/sag-1903-225.

45. Müzeyyen Yıldırım et al., "Preventing Cisplatin Induced Ototoxicity by N-Acetylcysteine and Salicylate," *Kulak Burun Bogaz Ihtisas Dergisi [Journal of Ear, Nose, and Throat]* 20, no. 4 (2010): 173–83, https://pubmed.ncbi.nlm.nih.gov/20626325.

46. Jie Deng et al., "N-Acetylcysteine Decreases Malignant."

47. Anselm Chi-wai Lee and LeLe Aung, "Treatment of Hepatic Veno-Occlusive Disease in Children with N-Acetylcysteine," *Pediatric Blood & Cancer* 66, no. 2 (2018): e27518, https://doi.org/10.1002/pbc.27518.

48. Lourdes Alvarez-Arellano et al., "Neuroprotective Effects of Quercetin in Pediatric Neurological Diseases," *Molecules* 25, no. 23 (2020): 5597, https://doi.org/10.3390/molecules25235597; Parisa Maleki Dana et al., "Anti-Cancer Properties of Quercetin in Osteosarcoma," *Cancer Cell International* 21, no. 1 (2021), https://doi.org/10.1186/s12935-021-02067-8.

49. Saleh A. Almatroodi et al., "Potential Therapeutic Targets of Quercetin, a Plant Flavonol, and Its Role in the Therapy of Various Types of Cancer through the Modulation of Various Cell Signaling Pathways," *Molecules* 26, no. 5 (2021): 1315, https://doi.org/10.3390/molecules26051315.

50. Liwei Wu et al., "Quercetin Shows Anti-Tumor Effect in Hepatocellular Carcinoma LM3 Cells by Abrogating JAK2/STAT3 Signaling Pathway," *Cancer Medicine* 8, no. 10 (2019): 4806–20, https://doi.org/10.1002/cam4.2388.

51. Himakshi Sidhar and Ranjit K. Giri, "Induction of *Bex* Genes by Curcumin Is Associated with Apoptosis and Activation of P53 in N2a Neuroblastoma Cells," *Scientific Reports* 7, (2017), https://doi.org/10.1038/srep41420.

52. Nicola Bortel et al., "Effects of Curcumin in Pediatric Epithelial Liver Tumors: Inhibition of Tumor Growth and Alpha-Fetoprotein *In Vitro* and *In Vivo* Involving the NFkappaB- and the Beta-Catenin Pathways," *Oncotarget* 6, no. 38 (2015): 40680–91, https://doi.org/10.18632/oncotarget.5673.

53. Bortel et al., "Effects of Curcumin."

54. Steven Johnson and Nasha Winters, *Mistletoe and the Emerging Future of Integrative Oncology* (Hudson, NY: Portal Books, 2021).

55. Julie Tabiasco, "Mistletoe Viscotoxins Increase Natural Killer Cell-Mediated Cytotoxicity," *European Journal of Biochemistry* 269, no. 10 (2002): 2591–600, https://doi.org/10.1046/j.1432-1033.2002.02932.x.

56. Seema Patel and Suryakanta Panda, "Emerging Roles of Mistletoes in Malignancy Management," *3 Biotech* 4, no. 1 (2014): 13–20, https://doi.org/10.1007/s13205-013-0124-6.

57. Alessandra Longhi et al., "A Randomized Study on Postrelapse Disease-Free Survival with Adjuvant Mistletoe versus Oral Etoposide in Osteosarcoma Patients," *Evidence-Based Complementary and Alternative Medicine* (2014): 1–9, https://doi.org/10.1155/2014/210198.

58. Franziska Böttger et al., "High-Dose Intravenous Vitamin C, a Promising Multi-Targeting Agent in the Treatment of Cancer," *Journal of Experimental & Clinical Cancer Research* 40, no. 1 (2021), https://doi.org/10.1186/s13046-021-02134-y.

59. Paul S. Anderson, "Intravenous Vitamin C in Naturopathic Oncology," presentation to the Oncology Association of Naturopathic Physicians, Scottsdale, Arizona, 2012; Paul S. Anderson, E. Naydis, and L. Standish, "High Dose IV Ascorbic Acid Therapy: The Bastyr Experience," poster session presented at the Society for Integrative Oncology, Cleveland, Ohio, November 2011.

60. Wolfgang Ferbiger et al., "*In Vitro* Cytotoxicity of Novel Platinum-Based Drugs and Dichloroacetate against Lung Carcinoid Cell Lines," *Clinical and Translational Oncology* 13 (2011): 43–49, https://doi.org/10.1007/s12094-011-0615-z; Edward B. Garon et al., "Dichloroacetate Should Be Considered with Platinum-Based Chemotherapy in Hypoxic Tumors Rather than as a Single Agent in Advanced Non–Small Cell Lung Cancer," *Journal of Cancer Research and Clinical Oncology* 140, no. 3 (2014): 443–52, https://doi.org/10.1007/s00432-014-1583-9.

61. E. M. Dunbar et al., "Phase 1 Trial of Dichloroacetate (DCA) in Adults with Recurrent Malignant Brain Tumors," *Investigational New Drugs* 32, no. 3 (2014): 452–64, https://doi.org/10.1007/s10637-013-0047-4; Laura Korsakova, Jan Aleksander Krasko, and Edgaras Stankevicius, "Metabolic-Targeted Combination Therapy with Dichloroacetate and Metformin Suppresses Glioblastoma Cell Line Growth *In Vitro* and *In Vivo*," *In Vivo* 35, no. 1 (2021): 341–48, https://doi.org/10.21873/invivo.12265.

62. Ravindran Kalathil Veena et al., "Antitumor Effects of Palladium–α–Lipoic Acid Complex Formulation as an Adjunct in Radiotherapy," *Journal of Environmental Pathology, Toxicology and Oncology* 35, no. 4 (2016): 333–42, https://doi.org/10.1615/JEnvironPatholToxicolOncol.2016016640.

63. Nicole J. Kubat, John Moffett, and Linley M. Fray, "Effect of Pulsed Electromagnetic Field Treatment on Programmed Resolution of Inflammation Pathway Markers in Human Cells in Culture," *Journal of Inflammation Research* 8 (2015): 59–69, https://doi.org/10.2147/JIR.S78631; Alex W. Thomas et al., "A Randomized, Double-Blind, Placebo-Controlled Clinical Trial Using a Low-Frequency Magnetic Field in the Treatment of Musculoskeletal Chronic Pain," *Pain Research & Management* 12, no. 4 (2007): 249–58, https://doi.org/10.1155/2007/626072; Shin-Hong Chen et al., "The Effect of Electromagnetic Field on Sleep of Patients with Nocturia," *Medicine* 101, no. 32 (2022): e29129, https://doi.org/10.1097/MD.0000000000029129; Glenn M. Stewart et al., "Impact of Pulsed Electromagnetic Field Therapy on Vascular Function and Blood Pressure in Hypertensive Individuals," *Journal of Clinical Hypertension* 22, no. 6 (2020): 1083–89, https://doi.org/10.1111/jch.13877; Kerstin Hug and Martin Röösli, "Therapeutic Effects of Whole-Body Devices Applying Pulsed Electromagnetic Fields (PEMF): A Systematic Literature Review," *Bioelectromagnetics* 33, no. 2 (2011): 95–105, https://doi.org/10.1002/bem.20703.

64. Sussanna Czeranko, "A Century After the Spanish Flu," *Naturopathic Doctor News & Review*, April 4, 2018, https://ndnr.com/nature-cure/a-century-after-the-spanish-flu.

65. Frank W. Stahnisch and Marja Verhoef, "The Flexner Report of 1910 and Its Impact on Complementary and Alternative Medicine and Psychiatry in North America in the 20th Century," *Evidence-Based Complementary and Alternative Medicine* (2012): 647896, https://doi.org/10.1155/2012/647896.

66. Quoc-Chuong Bui et al., "The Efficacy of Hyperbaric Oxygen Therapy in the Treatment of Radiation-Induced Late Side Effects," *International Journal of Radiation Oncology, Biology, Physics* 60, no. 3 (2004): 871–78, https://doi.org/10.1016/j.ijrobp.2004.04.019.
67. Bernardino Clavo et al., "Effects of Ozone Treatment on Health-Related Quality of Life and Toxicity Induced by Radiotherapy and Chemotherapy in Symptomatic Cancer Survivors," *International Journal of Environmental Research and Public Health* 20, no. 2 (2023): 1479, https://doi.org/10.3390/ijerph20021479.
68. U. Tirelli et al., "Oxygen-Ozone Therapy as Support and Palliative Therapy in 50 Cancer Patients with Fatigue—A Short Report," *European Review for Medical and Pharmacological Sciences* 22, no. 22 (2018): 8030–33, https://doi.org/10.26355/eurrev_201811_16432.
69. Vural Kesik et al., "Ozone Ameliorates Methotrexate-Induced Intestinal Injury in Rats," *Cancer Biology & Therapy* 8, no. 17 (2009): 1623–28, https://doi.org/10.4161/cbt.8.17.9203.
70. "Infrared Sauna Therapy and Its Effect on Cancer Cells?" Immunity Therapy Center, accessed June 20, 2022, https://www.immunitytherapycenter.com/blog/infrared-sauna-therapy-and-its-effect-on-cancer-cells.
71. Joy Hussain and Marc Cohen, "Clinical Effects of Regular Dry Sauna Bathing: A Systematic Review," *Evidence-Based Complementary and Alternative Medicine* 2018, https://doi.org/10.1155/2018/1857413.
72. Michael R. Hamblin, "Mechanisms and Applications of the Anti-Inflammatory Effects of Photobiomodulation," *AIMS Biophysics* 4, no. 3 (2017): 337–61, https://doi.org/10.3934/biophy.2017.3.337.
73. Daniëlle E. J. Starreveld et al., "Light Therapy for Cancer-Related Fatigue in (Non-)Hodgkin Lymphoma Survivors: Results of a Randomized Controlled Trial," *Cancers* 13, no. 19 (2021): 4948, https://doi.org/10.3390/cancers13194948; Judith A. E. M. Zecha et al., "Low Level Laser Therapy/Photobiomodulation in the Management of Side Effects of Chemoradiation Therapy in Head and Neck Cancer: Part 1: Mechanisms of Action, Dosimetric, and Safety Considerations," *Supportive Care in Cancer* 24, no. 6 (2016): 2781–92, https://doi.org/10.1007/s00520-016-3152-z.
74. Rodrigo Crespo Mosca et al., "The Efficacy of Photobiomodulation Therapy in Improving Tissue Resilience and Healing of Radiation Skin Damage," *Photonics* 9, no. 1 (2022): 10, https://doi.org/10.3390/photonics9010010; "Light Therapy Fast-Tracks Healing of Skin Damage from Cancer Radiation Therapy," *ScienceDaily*, January 27, 2022, https://www.sciencedaily.com/releases/2022/01/220127104305.htm.
75. Nadia Birocco et al., "The Effects of Reiki Therapy on Pain and Anxiety in Patients Attending a Day Oncology and Infusion Services Unit," *American Journal of Hospice and Palliative Medicine* 29, no. 4 (2011): 290–94, https://doi.org/10.1177/1049909111420859.

Chapter 8. Evaluate Cancer-Specific Integrative Therapies

1. Martin Belson, Beverly Kingsley, and Adrianne Holmes, "Risk Factors for Acute Leukemia in Children: A Review," *Environmental Health Perspectives* 115, no. 1 (2006): 138–45, https://doi.org/10.1289/ehp.9023; Andrew S. Park et al., "Prenatal Pesticide Exposure and Childhood Leukemia—A California Statewide Case-Control Study," *International Journal of Hygiene and Environmental Health* 226 (2020): 113486, https://doi.org/10.1016/j.ijheh.2020.113486; Felix M. Onyije et al., "Environmental Risk Factors for Childhood Acute Lymphoblastic Leukemia: An Umbrella Review," *Cancers* 14, no. 2 (2022): 382, https://doi.org/10.3390/cancers14020382.

2. Cancer Research UK, "Survival Statistics for Acute Lymphoblastic Leukaemia (ALL)," October 11, 2021, https://www.cancerresearchuk.org/about-cancer/acute-lymphoblastic-leukaemia-all/survival.

3. Matthew Tcheng et al., "Very Long Chain Fatty Acid Metabolism Is Required in Acute Myeloid Leukemia," *Blood* 137, no. 25 (2021): 3518–32, https://doi.org/10.1182/blood.2020008551.

4. Luis Rodriguez, "What Are the Most Common Childhood Brain Tumors?—On Call for All Kids," Johns Hopkins All Children's Hospital, YouTube video, April 5, 2021, https://www.youtube.com/watch?v=k6se3sX2AlM.

5. Chan Chung et al., "Integrated Metabolic and Epigenomic Reprograming by H3K27M Mutations in Diffuse Intrinsic Pontine Gliomas," *Cancer Cell* 38, no. 3 (2020): 334–49.e9, https://doi.org/10.1016/j.ccell.2020.07.008.

6. T. J. Zuzak et al., "Paediatric Medulloblastoma Cells Are Susceptible to *Viscum album* (Mistletoe) Preparations," *Anticancer Research* 26, no. 5A (2006): 3485–92, https://ar.iiarjournals.org/content/26/5A/3485.

7. Sidharth Mahapatra and Mark J. Amsbaugh, *Medulloblastoma* (Treasure Island, FL: StatPearls Publishing, 2020), https://www.ncbi.nlm.nih.gov/books/NBK431069.

8. Thomas N. Seyfried et al., "Ketogenic Metabolic Therapy, without Chemo or Radiation, for the Long-Term Management of *IDH1*-Mutant Glioblastoma: An 80-Month Follow-Up Case Report," *Frontiers in Nutrition* 8 (2021): 682243, https://doi.org/10.3389/fnut.2021.682243.

9. Amir Zahra et al., "Consuming a Ketogenic Diet while Receiving Radiation and Chemotherapy for Locally Advanced Lung Cancer and Pancreatic Cancer: The University of Iowa Experience of Two Phase 1 Clinical Trials," *Radiation Research* 187, no. 6 (2017): 743–54, https://doi.org/10.1667/RR14668.1; B. G. Allen et al., "Enhancing Tumor Chemo-radio-sensitization using Ketogenic Diets," *International Journal of Radiation Oncology, Biology, Physics* 78, no. 3 (2010), https://doi.org/10.1016/j.ijrobp.2010.07.292.

10. J. Eduardo Rodriguez-Almaraz and Nicholas Butowski, "Therapeutic and Supportive Effects of Cannabinoids in Patients with Brain Tumors (CBD Oil and Cannabis)," *Current Treatment Options in Oncology* 24, no. 1 (2023): 30–44, https://doi.org/10.1007/s11864-022-01047-y.

11. American Cancer Society, "Key Statistics about Neuroblastoma," April 28, 2021, https://www.cancer.org/cancer/neuroblastoma/about/key-statistics.html.

12. Rangarirai Makuku et al., "The Role of Ketogenic Diet in the Treatment of Neuroblastoma," *Integrative Cancer Therapies* 22 (2023), https://doi.org/10.1177/15347354221150787.

13. Serena Vella et al., "Dichloroacetate Inhibits Neuroblastoma Growth by Specifically Acting Against Malignant Undifferentiated Cells," *International Journal of Cancer* 130, no. 7 (2011): 1484–93, https://doi.org/10.1002/ijc.26173.

14. Sepideh Aminzadeh, Anna Kowalczuk, and Arkadiusz Szterk, "Energy Metabolism in Neuroblastoma and Wilms Tumor," *Translational Pediatrics* 4, no. 1 (2015): 20–32, https://doi.org/10.3978/j.issn.2224-4336.2015.01.04.

15. American Cancer Society, "Key Statistics for Non-Hodgkin Lymphoma in Children," January 12, 2023, https://www.cancer.org/cancer/childhood-non-hodgkin-lymphoma/about/key-statistics.html.

16. Neil McKinney, *Naturopathic Oncology* (Victoria, BC: Liaison Press, 2020), 420.

17. McKinney, *Naturopathic Oncology*, 420.

18. American Cancer Society, "Key Statistics for Rhabdomyosarcoma," January 8, 2020, https://www.cancer.org/cancer/rhabdomyosarcoma/about/key-statistics.html.

19. Anna Szurpnicka, Anna Kowalczuk, and Arkadiusz Szterk, "Biological Activity of Mistletoe: In Vitro and in Vivo Studies and Mechanisms of Action," *Archives of Pharmacal Research* 43, no. 6 (2020): 593–629, https://doi.org/10.1007/s12272-020-01247-w; Rahel Mascha Stammer et al., "Synergistic Antitumour Properties of *viscumTT* in Alveolar Rhabdomyosarcoma," *Journal of Immunology Research* (2017): 4874280, https://doi.org/10.1155/2017/4874280.

20. Szurpnicka et al., "Biological Activity of Mistletoe"; Stammer et al., "Synergistic Antitumour Properties of *viscumTT*."

21. Longhi et al., "A Randomized Study on Postrelapse."

22. Susann Kleinsimon et al., "ViscumTT Induces Apoptosis and Alters IAP Expression in Osteosarcoma in Vitro and Has Synergistic Action When Combined with Different Chemotherapeutic Drugs," *BMC Complementary and Alternative Medicine* 17, no. 1 (2017): 26, https://doi.org/10.1186/s12906-016-1545-7.

23. National Cancer Institute, "Childhood Adrenocortical Carcinoma Treatment (PDQ®)– Patient Version," October 24, 2019, https://www.cancer.gov/types/adrenocortical /patient/child-adrenocortical-treatment-pdq.

Chapter 9. Manage Side Effects

1. McKinney, *Naturopathic Oncology*.

2. Sajib Chakraborty and Taibur Rahman, "The Difficulties in Cancer Treatment," *ecancer* 6, no. 16 (2012), https://doi.org/10.3332/ecancer.2012.ed16.

3. Graeme Morgan, Robyn Ward, and Michael Barton, "The Contribution of Cytotoxic Chemotherapy to 5-Year Survival in Adult Malignancies," *Clinical Oncology* 16, no. 8 (2004): 549–60, https://doi.org/10.1016/j.clon.2004.06.007.

4. Stefanie de Groot et al., "Effects of Short-Term Fasting on Cancer Treatment," *Journal of Experimental & Clinical Cancer Research* 38, no. 1 (2019), https://doi.org/10.1186/s13046-019-1189-9.

5. Amy Mone and Valerie Mehl, "Intravenous Mistletoe Extract Shows Promise as Cancer Therapy in Small Study," *The Hub*, February 23, 2023, https://hub.jhu.edu/2023/02/23 /mistletoe-extract-cancer-treatment-study; Mohsen Marvibaigi et al., "Preclinical and Clinical Effects of Mistletoe against Breast Cancer," *BioMed Research International* (2014): 785479, https://doi.org/10.1155/2014/785479.

6. Cedric F. Garland et al., "The Role of Vitamin D in Cancer Prevention," *American Journal of Public Health* 96, no. 2 (2006): 252–61, https://doi.org/10.2105/AJPH.2004.045260; Paulette D. Chandler et al., "Effect of Vitamin D₃ Supplements on Development of Advanced Cancer: A Secondary Analysis of the VITAL Randomized Clinical Trial," *JAMA Network Open* 3, no. 11 (2020): e2025850, https://doi.org/10.1001/jamanetworkopen.2020.25850.

7. Russell Martin, "Vitamin D," *Life Extension*, August 2023, https://www.lifeextension .com/magazine/2006/3/report_vitamind; Tulay Kus et al., "The Predictive Value of Vitamin D Follow-Up and Supplementation on Recurrence in Patients with Colorectal Cancer," *Future Oncology* 18, no. 18 (2022), https://doi.org/10.2217/fon-2021-1410.

8. Paul S. Anderson, "Intravenous Ascorbic Acid and Oncologic Agents," presentation to the Oncology Association of Naturopathic Physicians Second Annual Meeting, Phoenix, Arizona, February 2013, https://www.consultdranderson.com/wp-content/uploads /securepdfs/2020/12/6-Ascorbate-and-Oncologic-Therapies-2020.pdf.

9. Brianne R. O'Leary et al., "Pharmacological Ascorbate as an Adjuvant for Enhancing Radiation-Chemotherapy Responses in Gastric Adenocarcinoma," *Radiation Research* 189,

no. 5 (2018): 456–65, https://doi.org/10.1667/RR14978.1; Gina Nauman et al., "Systematic Review of Intravenous Ascorbate in Cancer Clinical Trials," *Antioxidants* 7, no. 7 (2018): 89, https://doi.org/10.3390/antiox7070089; Anitra C. Carr and John Cook, "Intravenous Vitamin C for Cancer Therapy—Identifying the Current Gaps in Our Knowledge," *Frontiers in Physiology* 9 (2018), https://www.frontiersin.org/articles/10.3389/fphys.2018.01182/full; Consult Dr. A, "Antioxidants in Oncology: Blog and Literature Review," Anderson Medical Group, 2016 https://www.consultdranderson.com/antioxidants-in-oncology; Yan Ma et al., "High-Dose Parenteral Ascorbate Enhanced Chemosensitivity of Ovarian Cancer and Reduced Toxicity of Chemotherapy," *Science Translational Medicine* 6, no. 222 (2014), https://stm.sciencemag.org/content/6/222/222ra18; Matthew S. Alexander et al., "Pharmacologic Ascorbate Reduces Radiation-Induced Normal Tissue Toxicity and Enhances Tumor Radiosensitization in Pancreatic Cancer," *Cancer Research* 78, no. 24 (2018), https://doi.org/10.1158/0008-5472.CAN-18-1680.

10. Neil McKinney, *Naturopathic Oncology.*

Chapter 10. Detoxify

1. S. H. Zahm and M. H. Ward, "Pesticides and Childhood Cancer," *Environmental Health Perspectives* 106, suppl 3 (1998): 893–908, https://doi.org/10.1289/ehp.98106893; Mark Weller, "There's Something in the Air, and It Causes Childhood Cancers," Californians for Pesticide Reform, December 2021, https://www.pesticidereform.org/wp-content/uploads/2021/12/FINAL-202111-CPR-Childhood-Cancer-v4.pdf; Environmental Working Group, "Study Links Childhood Cancer and In-Home Pesticide Use," September 28, 2015, https://www.ewg.org/news-insights/news-release/study-links-childhood-cancer-and-home-pesticide-use.

2. Irma Martha Medina-Díaz et al., "The Relationship between Cancer and Paraoxonase 1," *Antioxidants* 11, no. 4 (2022): 697, https://doi.org/10.3390/antiox11040697.

3. Nazzareno Ballatori et al., "Glutathione Dysregulation and the Etiology and Progression of Human Diseases," *Biological Chemistry* 390, no. 3 (2009): 191–214, https://doi.org/10.1515/BC.2009.033; Wen Luo et al., "Glutathione S-Transferases in Pediatric Cancer," *Frontiers in Oncology* 1 (2011), https://doi.org/10.3389/fonc.2011.00039; Luke Kennedy et al., "Role of Glutathione in Cancer: From Mechanisms to Therapies," *Biomolecules* 10, no. 10 (2020): 1429, https://doi.org/10.3390/biom10101429.

4. Mariapia Vairetti et al., "Changes in Glutathione Content in Liver Diseases: An Update," *Antioxidants* 10, no. 3 (2021): 364, https://doi.org/10.3390/antiox10030364.

5. Vairetti et al., "Changes in Glutathione Content."

6. Ibrahim El-Serafi et al., "The Effect of N-Acetyl-l-Cysteine (NAC) on Liver Toxicity and Clinical Outcome after Hematopoietic Stem Cell Transplantation" *Scientific Reports* 8, no. 1 (2018), https://doi.org/10.1038/s41598-018-26033-z.

7. Gregory D. Sepich-Poore et al., "The Microbiome and Human Cancer," *Science* 371, no. 6536 (2021): eabc4552, https://doi.org/10.1126/science.abc4552; Julie M. Deleemans et al., "The Chemo-Gut Study: Investigating the Long-Term Effects of Chemotherapy on Gut Microbiota, Metabolic, Immune, Psychological and Cognitive Parameters in Young Adult Cancer Survivors: Study Protocol," *BMC Cancer* 19, no. 1 (2019): 1243, https://doi.org/10.1186/s12885-019-6473-8.

8. Patti Verbanas, "Antibiotic Exposure in Children under Age 2 Associated with Chronic Conditions," *Rutgers Today*, November 16, 2020, https://www.rutgers.edu/news/antibiotic-exposure-children-under-age-2-associated-chronic-conditions.

9. M. J. Arnaud, "Mild Dehydration: A Risk Factor of Constipation?" *European Journal of Clinical Nutrition* 57, suppl 2 (2003): S88–S95, https://doi.org/10.1038/sj.ejcn.1601907.

10. Aviva Romm, "Treating Children's Constipation Naturally: Move Over Miralax," February 4, 2015, https://avivaromm.com/7-steps-kids-constipation-naturally.

11. Debby Hamilton, "How to Protect Against Glyphosate Toxicity," *Townsend Letter*, accessed July 31, 2023, https://www.townsendletter.com/article/441-protect-against-glyphosate-toxicity.

12. Michelle Vallet, "Updates in Research: Manual Lymphatic Drainage," American Massage Therapy Association, May 1, 2023, https://www.amtamassage.org/publications/massage-therapy-journal/research-update-lymph-drainage.

13. Marc A. Russo, Danielle M. Santarelli, and Dean O'Rourke, "The Physiological Effects of Slow Breathing in the Healthy Human," *Breathe* 13, no. 4 (2017): 298–309, https://doi.org/10.1183/20734735.009817.

14. S. H. Zahm and M. H. Ward, "Pesticides and Childhood Cancer"; "Pesticides Linked to Adult and Childhood Cancer in Western U.S., with Incidence Varying by County," *Beyond Pesticides Daily News Blog*, June 28, 2022, https://beyondpesticides.org/dailynewsblog/2022/06/pesticides-linked-to-adult-and-childhood-cancer-in-western-u-s-with-incidence-varying-by-county; Naveen Joseph et al., "Investigation of Relationships Between the Geospatial Distribution of Cancer Incidence and Estimated Pesticide Use in the U.S. West," *GeoHealth* 6, no. 5 (2022), https://doi.org/10.1029/2021GH000544; Naveen Joseph and Alan S. Kolok, "Assessment of Pediatric Cancer and Its Relationship to Environmental Contaminants: An Ecological Study in Idaho," *GeoHealth* 6, no. 3 (2022), https://doi.org/10.1029/2021GH000548; Mei Chen et al., "Residential Exposure to Pesticide During Childhood and Childhood Cancers: A Meta-Analysis," *Pediatrics* 136, no. 4 (2015): 719–29, https://doi.org/10.1542/peds.2015-0006.

15. Hamilton, "How to Protect against Glyphosate Toxicity."

16. Henning Gerlach et al., "Oral Application of Charcoal and Humic Acids Influence Selected Gastrointestinal Microbiota, Enzymes, Electrolytes, and Substrates in the Blood of Dairy Cows Challenged with Glyphosate in GMO Feeds," *Journal of Environmental & Analytical Toxicology* 5, no. 2 (2014), https://doi.org/10.4172/2161-0525.1000256; "Glyphosate Toxicity in Cows Successfully Treated with Charcoal and Sauerkraut," *GM Watch*, January 15, 2015, https://www.gmwatch.org/en/106-news/latest-news/15875-glyphosate-toxicity-in-cows-successfully-treated-with-charcoal-and-sauerkraut.

17. Livio Pagano et al., "Risk Assessment and Prognostic Factors for Mould-Related Diseases in Immunocompromised Patients," *Journal of Antimicrobial Chemotherapy* 66, suppl. 1 (2011): i5–14, https://doi.org/10.1093/jac/dkq437.

18. Brice, "Moskowitz: Cellphone Radiation Is Harmful."

19. M. Nathaniel Mead, "Cancer: Strong Signal for Cell Phone Effects," *Environmental Health Perspectives* 116, no. 10 (2008): A422, https://doi.org/10.1289/ehp.116-a422; "Meta-Analysis Shows Increased Risk of Tumors for Cell Phone Users," *Berkeley Public Health*, December 15, 2020, https://publichealth.berkeley.edu/news-media/research-highlights/meta-analysis-shows-increased-risk-of-tumors-for-cell-phone-users.

20. "After Several Childhood Cancer Cases at One School, Parents Question Radiation from Cell Tower," *CBS News*, April 4, 2019, https://www.cbsnews.com/news/cell-tower-shut-down-some-california-parents-link-to-several-cases-of-childhood-cancer.
21. Joy J. Chebet et al., "Effect of D-Limonene and Its Derivatives on Breast Cancer in Human Trials: A Scoping Review and Narrative Synthesis," *BMC Cancer* 21, no. 1 (2021): 902, https://doi.org/10.1186/s12885-021-08639-1.
22. Xin Jiang et al., "Chemopreventive Activity of Sulforaphane," *Drug Design, Development and Therapy* 12 (2018): 2905–13, https://doi.org/10.2147/DDDT.S100534.
23. Suhaniza Sulaiman et al., "Chemopreventive Effect of *Chlorella vulgaris* in Choline Deficient Diet and Ethionine Induced Liver Carcinogenesis in Rats," *International Journal of Cancer Research* 2, no. 3 (2006): 234–41, https://doi.org/10.3923/ijcr.2006.234.241.
24. Siddavaram Nagini, Fabrizio Palitti, and Adayapalam T. Natarajan, "Chemopreventive Potential of Chlorophyllin: A Review of the Mechanisms of Action and Molecular Targets," *Nutrition and Cancer* 67, no. 2 (2015): 203–11, https://doi.org/10.1080/01635581.2015.990573.

Chapter 11. Restore the Gut

1. Deleemans et al., "The Chemo-Gut Study"; "Late Effects of Treatment for Childhood Cancer (PDQ®)–Health Professional Version," National Cancer Institute, September 11, 2023, https://www.cancer.gov/types/childhood-cancers/late-effects-hp-pdq.
2. "What Are the Late Effects of Childhood Cancer?" Cancer.Net, October 2022, https://www.cancer.net/navigating-cancer-care/children/late-effects-childhood-cancer.
3. Deleemans et al., "The Chemo-Gut Study."
4. Jay Furst, "Study Finds Antibiotics before Age 2 Associated with Childhood Health Issues," *Mayo Clinic News Network*, November 16, 2020, https://newsnetwork.mayoclinic.org/discussion/study-finds-antibiotics-before-age-2-associated-with-childhood-health-issues.
5. Andrea Pession et al., "Fecal Microbiota Transplantation in Allogeneic Hematopoietic Stem Cell Transplantation Recipients: A Systematic Review," *Journal of Personalized Medicine* 11, no. 2 (2021): 100, https://doi.org/10.3390/jpm11020100; "Fecal Transplants Boost Helpful Microbiota for Stem Cell Transplant Patients," Memorial Sloan Kettering Cancer Center, April 1, 2022, https://www.mskcc.org/news/gut-check-microbiota-and-its-role.
6. "Fecal Transplants Boost Helpful Microbiota."
7. Florent Malard, Xiao-Jun Huang, and Joycelyn P. Y. Sim, "Treatment and Unmet Needs in Steroid-Refractory Acute Graft-Versus-Host Disease," *Leukemia* 34, no. 5 (2020): 1229–40, https://doi.org/10.1038/s41375-020-0804-2.
8. "Fecal Transplants Help Patients with Advanced Melanoma Respond to Immunotherapy," National Cancer Institute, February 4, 2021, https://www.cancer.gov/news-events/press-releases/2021/fecal-transplants-cancer-immunotherapy; Jie Zhang et al., "Cancer Immunotherapy: Fecal Microbiota Transplantation Brings Light," *Current Treatment Options in Oncology* 23, no. 12 (2022): 1777–92, https://doi.org/10.1007/s11864-022-01027-2.

Chapter 12. Heal the Child, Heal the Family

1. Astri Syse et al., "Does Childhood Cancer Affect Parental Divorce Rates? A Population-Based Study," *Journal of Clinical Oncology* 28, no. 5 (2010): 872–77, https://doi.org/10.1200/JCO.2009.24.0556.

2. Craig Erker et al., "Impact of Pediatric Cancer on Family Relationships," *Cancer Medicine* 7, no. 5 (2018): 1680–88, https://doi.org/10.1002/cam4.1393.

3. Josymar Chacin-Fernández et al., "Psychological Intervention Based on Psychoneuroimmunology Improves Clinical Evolution, Quality of Life, and Immunity of Children with Leukemia: A Preliminary Study," *Health Psychology Open* 6, no. 1 (2019), https://doi.org/10.1177/2055102919838902.

4. "Evidence Mounts for Link between Opioids and Cancer Growth," UChicago Medicine, March 20, 2012, https://www.uchicagomedicine.org/forefront/news/evidence-mounts-for-link-between-opioids-and-cancer-growth.

5. Adrian Szczepaniak, Jakub Fichna, and Marta Zielińska, "Opioids in Cancer Development, Progression and Metastasis: Focus on Colorectal Cancer," *Current Treatment Options in Oncology* 21, no. 1 (2020), https://doi.org/10.1007/s11864-019-0699-1.

6. Autumn M. Gallegos et al., "Meditation and Yoga for Posttraumatic Stress Disorder: A Meta-Analytic Review of Randomized Controlled Trials," *Clinical Psychology Review* 58 (2017): 115–24, https://doi.org/10.1016/j.cpr.2017.10.004; Erica Edwards, "Meditation as Effective as Medication for Anxiety, Study Finds," *NBC News*, November 9, 2022, https://www.nbcnews.com/health/health-news/meditation-effective-medication-anxiety-study-finds-rcna56164; "How Meditation Helps with Depression," *Harvard Health Publishing*, August 1, 2018, https://www.health.harvard.edu/mind-and-mood/how-meditation-helps-with-depression.

7. Alice G. Walton, "Science Shows Meditation Benefits Children's Brains and Behavior," *Forbes*, October 18, 2016, https://www.forbes.com/sites/alicegwalton/2016/10/18/the-many-benefits-of-meditation-for-children.

8. Emma M. Seppälä et al., "Breathing-Based Meditation Decreases Posttraumatic Stress Disorder Symptoms in U.S. Military Veterans: A Randomized Controlled Longitudinal Study," *Journal of Traumatic Stress* 27, no. 4 (2014): 397–405, https://doi.org/10.1002/jts.21936.

9. Jennifer Aleman, "Reiki Provides Relaxation Treatment to Those with PTSD," *Hope for the Warriors*, https://www.hopeforthewarriors.org/reiki-provides-relaxation-treatment-to.

10. Giulia Zucchetti et al., "The Power of Reiki: Feasibility and Efficacy of Reducing Pain in Children with Cancer Undergoing Hematopoietic Stem Cell Transplantation," *Journal of Pediatric Oncology Nursing* 36, no. 5 (2019): 361–68, https://doi.org/10.1177/1043454219845879.

11. Li, "Effect of Forest Bathing Trips."

12. K. Chandrasekhar et al., "A Prospective, Randomized Double-Blind, Placebo-Controlled Study of Safety and Efficacy of a High-Concentration Full-Spectrum Extract of Ashwagandha Root in Reducing Stress and Anxiety in Adults," *Indian Journal of Psychological Medicine* 34, no. 3 (2012): 255–62, https://doi.org/10.4103/0253-7176.106022.

13. Laura Jones, "Nervines and Adaptogens: Naturopathic Choices for Anxiety, Stress and the Nervous System," *Whole Health Concord*, June 22, 2019, https://naturalmedicinenh.com/2019/06/22/nervines-and-adaptogens-naturopathic-choices-for-anxiety-stress-the-nervous-system.

14. Jordan Fallis, "13 Proven Ways Saunas Can Improve Your Mental Health," *Optimal Living Dynamics*, October 17, 2023, https://www.optimallivingdynamics.com/blog/13-proven-ways-saunas-can-improve-your-mental-health-dry-hot-benefits-depression-anxiety.

15. Ashley E. Mason et al., "Feasibility and Acceptability of a Whole-Body Hyperthermia (WBH) Protocol," *International Journal of Hyperthermia* 38, no. 1 (2021): 1529–35, https://doi.org/10.1080/02656736.2021.1991010.
16. Franklin King IV and Rebecca Hammond, "Psychedelics as Reemerging Treatments for Anxiety Disorders: Possibilities and Challenges in a Nascent Field," *Focus* 19, no. 2 (2021): 190–96, https://doi.org/10.1176/appi.focus.20200047.
17. Gabrielle Agin-Liebes and Alan K. Davis, "Psilocybin for the Treatment of Depression: A Promising New Pharmacotherapy Approach," *Current Topics in Behavioral Neurosciences* 56 (2021): 125–40, https://doi.org/10.1007/7854_2021_282.
18. Joseph M. Rootman et al., "Adults Who Microdose Psychedelics Report Health Related Motivations and Lower Levels of Anxiety and Depression Compared to Non-Microdosers," *Scientific Reports* 11, no. 1 (2021): 22479, https://doi.org/10.1038/s41598-021-01811-4.
19. Jennifer Chen, "How New Ketamine Drug Helps with Depression," *Yale Medicine*, March 21, 2019, https://www.yalemedicine.org/news/ketamine-depression.

Appendix A. Interpreting Test Results

1. Arnoud J. Templeton et al., "Prognostic Role of Neutrophil-to-Lymphocyte Ratio in Solid Tumors: A Systematic Review and Meta-Analysis," *Journal of the National Cancer Institute* 106, no. 6 (2014), https://doi.org/10.1093/jnci/dju124.
2. Digant Gupta and Christopher G. Lis, "Pretreatment Serum Albumin as a Predictor of Cancer Survival: A Systematic Review of the Epidemiological Literature," *Nutrition Journal* 9, no. 69 (2010), https://doi.org/10.1186/1475-2891-9-69.

Index

cannabinoids, individualized treatment with, 82–83

cannabis oil
  for chemotherapy side effects, 82, 114–15, 121, 123, 125
  for surgery-related pain, 156

carbohydrates
  in grains and legumes, 63
  ketosis stimulated by reducing, 68
  in Level 1 Nutrition, 68
  in Level 2 Nutrition, 69–70

carbon dioxide blood tests, 175

carcinogens
  common, 48
  early childhood exposure to, 47–51
  in food, 59

cardiac toxicity, integrative support for, 123

Carsyn Neille Foundation, 199

CAR T clinical trial, 164–65

castor oil packs, for liver support, 130–31

CBC (complete blood count) tests, 24, 25, 169–173

CBD (cannabidiol)
  for chemotherapy side effects, 114–15
  individualized treatment with, 82, 83
  for pain, 156
  for stress management, 160
  supplier for, 197

Cellcore, 138

central nervous system tumors
  brain tumors, 71, 76, 95, 100–101
  spinal cord tumors, 100–101

cesarean section birth, microbiome influenced by, 51, 56

charcoal, as binder, 134

Charlie Foundation for Ketogenic Therapies, 195

chemotherapy
  cannabinoids for, 82, 114–15, 121, 123, 125
  detoxification from, 138–39
  fasting benefits, 47, 72, 112–13
  general integrative support for, 112–15

  gut health role in effectiveness of, 52
  integrative support for side effects from, 120–27
  integrative support for specific types of, 115–19
  movement therapy for, 80
  overview, 111–12
  short-term fasting during, 47
  toxicity of, 115, 130

chest compression, for respiratory support, 136

chlorella and chlorophyll, for detoxification, 142

circadian rhythm disruption
  basic therapies for, 79
  stress from, 58

circulating tumor cell (CTC) tests, 36

Clean Fifteen fruits and vegetables, 61

clinical trials, supporting your child during, 107

clinicians. *See* metabolic oncology practitioners

Clostridioides difficile infections, fecal transplants for, 150

clothing, carcinogens in, 49–50

CMP (comprehensive metabolic panel) tests, 24, 25–26, 173–77

cognitive-behavioral therapy, 157

cognitive impairment, integrative support for, 121

complete blood count (CBC) tests, 24, 25, 169–173

comprehensive metabolic panel (CMP) tests, 24, 25–26, 173–77

computed tomography scans. *See* CT (computed tomography) scans

COMT SNPs, 57

constipation
  digestive support for, 134
  integrative support for, 121
  from ketosis, 71

constipation
  magnesium for, 70

consumer products, toxins in, 50

contrast agents, in imaging, 30, 32

About the Author

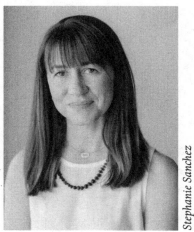

Stephanie Sanchez

DAGMARA BEINE HOLDS A PhD IN INTEGRATIVE MEDICINE, HAS over a decade of experience as a certified physician's assistant in emergency medicine, and is the founder, CEO, and clinical practitioner at her Wisconsin-based integrative health clinic, Zuza's Way. Motivated by her daughter Zuza's multiple fights against acute myeloid leukemia (AML) and a steadfast belief that there is a better way than what conventional oncology can offer, Dr. Beine changed her medical direction from emergency medicine to integrative oncology and developed a holistic, terrain-based approach to treating her patients. She is a graduate of Dr. Nasha Winters's Physician Mastermind program, Dr. Aviva Romm's Women's Integrative and Functional Medicine Certification Program, and the Kresser Institute's ADAPT Functional Medicine Practitioner Certification Program. Dr. Beine resides with her family in Wisconsin.

About the Foreword Authors

Dr. Nasha Winters, ND, La.C., FABNO, is the executive director of the Metabolic Institute of Health and co-author of *The Metabolic Approach to Cancer* and *Mistletoe and the Emerging Future of Integrative Oncology*.

A nationally recognized educator and clinician, Dr. Paul Anderson, NMD, is the founder of numerous clinics specializing in the treatment of cancer. He is the coauthor of *Outside the Box Cancer Therapies* and the author of *Cancer: The Journey from Diagnosis to Empowerment*.

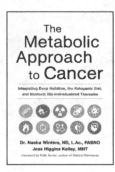
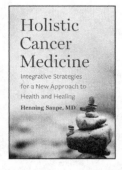
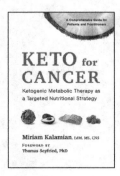
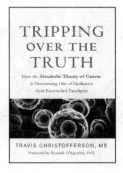
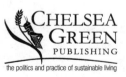

the politics and practice of sustainable living

CHELSEA GREEN PUBLISHING

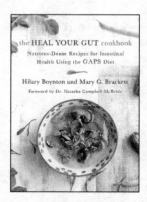

THE HEAL YOUR GUT COOKBOOK
Nutrient-Dense Recipes for Intestinal Health
Using the GAPS Diet
HILARY BOYNTON AND MARY G. BRACKETT
9781603585613
Paperback

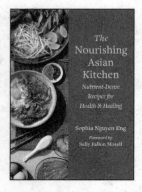

THE NOURISHING ASIAN KITCHEN
Nutrient-Dense Recipes for Health and Healing
SOPHIA NGUYEN ENG
9781645022169
Paperback

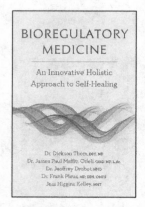

BIOREGULATORY MEDICINE
An Innovative Holistic Approach to Self-Healing
DICKSON THOM, JAMES PAUL MAFFITT ODELL,
JEOFFREY DROBOT, FRANK PLEUS,
AND JESS HIGGINS KELLEY
9781603588218
Paperback

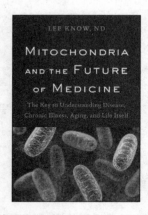

MITOCHONDRIA AND THE FUTURE OF MEDICINE
The Key to Understanding Disease, Chronic Illness,
Aging, and Life Itself
LEE KNOW
9781603587679
Paperback

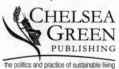

the politics and practice of sustainable living

For more information,
visit **www.chelseagreen.com**.